Seasons of Mirrors:
Consecration Leads to Revelation

by

LeShaun M. Taylor

Seasons of Mirrors: Consecration Leads to Revelation

(c) 2019 LeShaun M. Taylor

www.leshauntaylor.com

ISBN 978-1-944155-22-3

Library of Congress Control Number 2019905657

Seasons of Mirrors is published by Jozef PA of Louisiana LLC under the Jozef Syndicate imprint. For information, write to P.O. Box 318013, Baton Rouge, LA, 70831. Editing by Candace J. Semien. www.jozefsyndicate.com. Cover design by T. Jones Media and Traneisha Jones,

Printed in the United States of America

40th Birthday and Forty Days

The birthing of this book began in 2009 when God began dealing with me about starting a forty-day consecration on my fortieth birthday. I was not in a good place in my life nor in my relationship with God and I wanted, no wait, I needed to be closer to Him. At that time, I was the full-time caretaker for my mother who had recently had a massive stroke which left her paralyzed. I had my teenage daughter, no stable church home, and a part-time job which limited what I could do for my daughter.

When God led me to write this book to share with my daughter and then generations to come, I was excited. When He said this will be a book for all people I said "what you talking about Lord"! I questioned, "Why me, Lord?" However, I said "yes" to the Lord and now, friend, you hold within your hands my very first literary work. While on this consecration I received revelation, real answers, and clarity from God about myself.

The revelations that you are about to read are not in order of time but according to how the Holy Spirit led me through the consecrated forty days. These pages were written as directed by God to provide you with a snapshot of various situations I found myself in. Therefore, the flow in age or time will be a journey of life experiences, coupled with scriptures and truth regarding each situation. This is a transparent book that reveals all of my insecurities, fears, failures, and disappointments. It details my self-destructive behavior which I experienced throughout my life.

I used to find myself in a place of pity and sorrow—over and over again! That feeling had been such a significant part of my life for so long, until I deemed it my third eye. Even now, I sit here reminiscing over my life, trying to figure out when did I open myself up to allow schemes of the devil to make me feel like I belonged to him and not God. I realize now that there are so many women who feel the same way: burned out and scarred. It seems like only yesterday that I was one of those women. Thankfully, today, I am not.

On this journey of self-evaluation, I am learning to accept responsibility for my failures, bad decisions, hurts received and caused. Even when I knew the way of truth, I chose disobedience and the world's way of living. Yes, this was the beginning of my Seasons of Mirrors.

Just like an alcoholic has to admit there is a problem before they can ever start at a hint of a recovery process, we have to admit to them as well. I learned this from my dear friend who is now a proud recovered alcoholic. Now, here I am admitting that I may have to give more credit to myself for my mess, than even the devil!

Against You, You only, have I sinned and done what is evil in Your sight.

Psalm 51:4, NIV

Prayer
I am not a perfect person but you are a perfect God. I thank You for loving me in spite of my wicked ways. I don't always act as I should; pray as I should, give or forgive as I should, but You are yet faithful. Your grace and mercy forever covers me. Yes even in my ignorance, You yet cover me. I thank You, Lord God, for never changing, even when I do.

With much love,
Your daughter

These forty days would be more challenging than I could have ever imagined. I knew that not watching television and not eating would be hard but the greatest struggle for me was ALL spiritual.

God purged me dry! Every day of the consecration, he revealed me to me. From hidden anger, suppressed hurt to the fact that I never really got over being molested as a child. But he dealt with me in the area I struggled with the most ALL things sexual. From defiling my marriage bed to masturbation and oral sex.

Yes, the mirror God placed before me would be a hard one to look in. The consecration started with God instructing me to write down the names of everyone I had been sexually connected including those who shared "even a little" phone sex. Yes, He said write them ALL down. I didn't realize what He was stirring in me but when He finished I never looked at the gift of me, my body, my soul the same. I am most grateful and now I share what I have learned.

Seasons of Mirrors

One day, while I was at work, I started seeing myself in every person and situation that I was being judgmental about. If I looked at someone and thought, "Why she got those shoes on with that outfit?" Before I could finish the thought or comment, these interna mirrors would appear around me so that I could see nothing but myself. The first couple of times this happened I was like, "Ok what in the world?" But the more the mirrors appeared, the more I started looking closely at myself, judging myself, and being condescending to myself! It did not feel good. I did not look as good as I thought I did, inside or out.

The mirrors began to reveal the dirt and filth that laid dormant in my spirit! I saw hurts, pains, bitterness, anger, resentment and the deadliest one of all….unforgiveness. Once I began to seriously deal with these issues, then the mirrors would come only when I wanted to think a thought that was unbecoming or contrary to the word of God; stopping me in my tracks before I could even establish a negative thought.

Those mirrors were frightening but necessary. I began having more compassion for myself which I had never done before. More importantly, I began having compassion for other people and situations around me. The scripture is very clear:

> "Do not judge, or you too will be judged. For in the same way you judge others, you will be judged, and with the measure you use, it will be measured to you. "Why do you look at the speck of sawdust in your brother's eye and pay no attention to the plank in your own eye? How can you say to your brother, 'Let

me take the speck out of your eye,' when all the time there is a plank in your own eye? You hypocrite, first take the plank out of your own eye, and then you will see clearly to remove the speck from your brother's eye. "Do not give dogs what is sacred; do not throw your pearls to pigs. If you do, they may trample them under their feet, and turn and tear you to pieces.

Matthew 7:1-6, NIV

If we are to be judged, it should be by God and not each other. My seasons of mirrors showed me that yes, it was me all along! Whether someone loved, liked, barely liked, or even hated the ground that I walked on, which by the way belongs to God, it still gives me no right to judge, talk about, or belittle God's people. Now, I thank God for those mirrors that seem to pop up when I needed to see my true self and sometimes these mirrors were just to clearly remind me of how far I was away from God but still cloaked in His protection.

The teachers of the law and the Pharisees brought in a woman caught in adultery. They made her stand before the group 4 and said to Jesus, "Teacher, this woman was caught in the act of adultery. In the Law Moses commanded us to stone such women. Now what do you say?" they were using this question as a trap, in order to have a basis for accusing him. But Jesus bent down and started to write on the ground with his finger. When they kept on questioning him, he straightened up and said to them, "If any one of you is without sin, let him be the first to throw a stone at her." Again, He stooped down and wrote on the ground. At this, those who heard began to go away one at a time, the older ones first, until only Jesus was left, with the woman still standing there. Jesus straightened up and asked her, "Woman, where are they? Has no one condemned you?" "No one, sir," she said. "Then neither do I condemn you," Jesus declared. "Go now and leave your life of sin."

John 8:3-11, NIV

Writing Their Names

I wanted a closer walk with the Lord, up to this point my relationship with God was wishy-washy at best. I was unstable in all of my ways: from my spiritual walk, to my non-existent prayer life, my mental health, relationships both past and present, and my issues with all things fleshly. I prayed for God to cleanse me but while in the process reveal, purge, and deliver me. Well, I will say this, ask and it shall be given unto you whether you like it or not.

One subject that I started dealing with right away was sexual sin and the body. I thought this can't be too bad I just need to repent and move on but God had other plans. I was instructed to get a pen and some paper so I could write down the names of EVERY person I had been involved with in any way, shape or form in a sexual way. I stopped cold turkey, put the pen down and shouted,

"THE DEVIL!" I just sat there in awe trying to see how many sheets of paper I had. Yes, it was that serious for me and immediately I felt ashamed and did not want to write any of it in front of God—the same God who knew how many strands of hair I have on my head, the Almighty One, the Great Creator, I was ashamed and I hadn't even written down the first name.

I thought *why, Lord? How is this relevant?* Then, I was reminded this is what I prayed for. "You wanted revelation, you wanted deliverance, you wanted to be purged and that is exactly what we are going to do!"

I began to check myself. Was I strong enough for this? And I determined that I was! Then, I pressed forward and started with the very first name and then the next. Both were names of brothers who molested me as a child. I paused and realized they were pedophiles—something we rarely acknowledge.

Every night before bed I would tell myself, "Okay, Glad that's over" only to wake up the next morning with two or three names I had forgotten about or had buried deep down in my soul. I found myself writing as many as four names down every few days. When I had to flip the paper over to continue writing names, I cried out to God like never before. I repented and I cried some more. After a couple of weeks of writing the names of people I'd had sexual experiences with, I was exhausted but as I continued, I began to heal in areas that I didn't realize were hurting. Honestly, I thought I was already over those experiences.

I have attended church since I was about six years old. So, accordingly, I am one of the ones who can vaunt the age-old cliché, "I grew up in the church!" And even though it is true, I cannot say that I ever really had a true understanding of God, Jesus, or the church. I just knew that I loved being in church. There I felt a sense of security; like I belonged and was appreciated for being me: the talkative, strong willed, visionary, zealous me! However, as I got older and my life grew to be more and more of a mess, I learned how to balance the world and the church. I was able to maintain my sinful nature while drinking till drunk, smoking weed and cigarettes, selling drugs, being promiscuous and so much more. I believed that as long as I go to church I am doing my part to ensure my place in heaven. I remember when I finally asked the Lord into my heart. I was tired, drained and exhausted with life and myself. I wanted to be used of God. So, I began to seek His face and cry out to Him in sheer pain asking him, "Lord, why am I here, what do you really need with me? I feel as though I have no true value or worth. I am just here wasting space." And I heard the following scripture:

'For I know the plans I have for you,' declares the Lord, 'plans to prosper you and not to harm you, plans to give you hope and a future.'

Jeremiah 29:11, NIV

That scripture really encouraged me. It blessed me so much so that I decided that I really wanted to use my gifts and talents for His glory. I then found this scripture:

> *Therefore, my beloved brethren, be ye steadfast, unmovable, always abounding in the work of the Lord, forasmuch as ye know that your labour is not in vain in the Lord.*
>
> *I Corinthians 15:58*

After learning these scriptures, I knew I had to make some real changes in my spiritual life and walk. I had to tell myself to stop going from church to church, state to state, job to job and relationship to relationship! As I desired more from God, I realized that I had never been stable enough, especially in ministry, to receive wisdom, knowledge or understanding. I often found things in my life to blame my ignorance on, but I had to be honest with myself enough to acknowledge that it was not the job, the church, or the failed relationships. It was me!

Revelation of Sexual Immorality

As I read and studied the Word of God, this is one of the first scriptures that God led me to:

Do you not know that your bodies are members of Christ himself? Shall I then take the members of Christ and unite them with a prostitute? Never! Do you not know that he who unites himself with a prostitute is one with her body for it is said that the two will become one flesh.
1 Corinthians 6:15-16, NIV

Paul's assertion, in this scripture, is that our bodies are the members of Christ. Our body is not only for the Lord, but it belongs to Him by virtue of his redemptive work on the cross. Because we, as believers in the gospel of Jesus Christ are united to Him, this union pertains not only to the soul, but also to our physical bodies. God also took me to these scriptures: 1 Corinthians. 12:27, Romans 8:6-11, Ephesians 6:2-7 (Please dedicate some time to read them also).

Because our physical bodies belong to the Lord, it is this fact above all else that makes fornication such a wicked, malicious act of sin. To this, Paul declares to us that God forbids such acts. He then goes on to expound on this point to say that he who is joined to a harlot is one body. The verb joined (Greek, kollao) is used in Genesis 2:24, regarding the relationship between husband and wife. It is also used to reference man's relationship to God in Deuteronomy 10:20, 11:22; Jeremiah 13:11. This is why we must understand the significance of our bodies and God's intentions for them.

I have dealt with and, in some cases, continue to pray against, several sexual immoral spirits. Some of those which have been revealed to me have been hard to swallow. We must never fool ourselves into believing that because we have accepted Jesus Christ, we are now above Satan's desire to tempt us with desires from our past. I have tried to down play those desires but in order for true deliverance to take place, I must take responsibility for these demonic spirits and the strongmen that are attached. Responsibility in calling them out, responsibility in canceling their assignments, responsibility in casting them out in the Holy name of Jesus Christ of Nazareth! All of this falls on my willingness to be truthful and real with myself first!

I realized that calling a demonic spirit out by name is good for casting it into outer darkness; however, we must understand where the root that gave him access resides. Where or from what circumstance did the demon originate? By defining the root, it brings clarity and understanding as well as the ability to release the demon of its legal right to reside there! God knows I need both clarity and understanding. I constantly ask Him to guide me into true supernatural knowledge of these spirits and purpose for which they exist, so that I can bind them and cast them out in order to fight through to find the me HE can see!

This List is Growing

I had absolutely no desire to continue writing this list or finishing these forty days. The memories, the reflections, the emotions were all too raw. Here I was looking at a list of men. I'd quickly written down the first names that came to mind. They were the names of my molesters. It took a few days for me to pick up the list again. I prayed and fasted for healing and release from this assignment. I didn't want to go to the beginning. Then, I saw teenagers and young girls around me who reflected my life and the memories returned.

Growing up as a child, rejection was a factor in me having so many emotionally charged and destructive relationships. I carried a spirit of hopelessness and believed that I had to cover up my hurts and pains with fake smiles and laughter. I held on to hurt, bitterness, anger, and unrealistic expectations of myself and others. I wanted so badly to pull something out of my dad that he never had to give. I wanted him to validate me, to cherish me, to make me feel good about myself. I carried that desire into so many wrong relationships with men. I tried repeatedly to make the person I was in relationship with change and understand and provide what I needed. I often conceded to them by thinking, *You may smoke a little drink a little, and it is even okay if you blacken my eye, bust my lip, and curse me out, because in the end I will change you.*

As I sat in this moment of consecration, I began truly reflecting and God allowed me to see my past clearly. When I was a little girl, my relationship with my father was not the very best it could have been. I felt that at times he did not like me, let alone love me. I was always a very talkative child. I always had something to say no matter what the conversation. My mouth never quite connected to my brain so I did not understand that silence is sometimes golden. I was so outspoken and believed I could say or do anything. I was very independent and bold in spirit and I am not sure if my dad liked that. I desperately needed him to be a father to me. I needed his love and respect, but most of all, I needed his approval. As a child, my need for him was more important than the air I breathed. We never really had a real father-daughter relationship. He was simply emotionally unavailable to me. I have never been able to go to Daddy and release any of my hurts, joys, or pains. To be honest, I never knew how significant the blow of not having him in my life would play a major part in my future until I reached my early thirties.

My mother, on the other hand, is the type of person who liked to please. She was the one who bent over backwards, always going above and beyond the call of duty for anyone. When I would come home from school with good grades, I would always run past my mom in order to reach my dad. I hoped that I would get a kind word, a pat on the back, or maybe even a kiss on the cheek, but that never happened. I wanted and needed what I felt only my dad could give. What was it really that I needed from my dad? I did not know for sure, but I knew that his "Yeah, that's good," carried more weight than any of my Mom's "Ooh, baby, I am so proud of you" or "You did a good job."

At one time in my life, I would have said that my father was a heartless man. I really thought he didn't love me. My mom has always told me that my dad did love me and that he showed that love the best way he knew how. I have never seen him cry, smile much, or even give a compliment. In my forty-one years of life, only once has he told me that he loves me. That was more than twenty-five years ago and yet I still yearn for the day I would hear it again.

The very first man who hit me and left a lasting impression on me was my Dad. I clearly remember that day. I was showering and Dad was shaving. Daddy used that stuff from back in the day—Magic Shave. While shaving, Dad said, "Don't forget to wash your face." Now, I thought that was the craziest thing to say to someone who was taking a shower. So I sucked my teeth in a way to say without saying, "Dog, what do you think I'm going to do in here?" Well, baby, I don't know even today how he found my face through a closed shower curtain, but he did. I felt an overwhelming blow to my face. As I looked down and saw blood dripping from my mouth to the drain, I knew I should not have done that.

Later that night, my mom came into my room and apologized for my dad's actions, totally ignoring my chipped tooth. She said, "He didn't mean to do it." She asked me if I was ok. Then she told me and my sister goodnight as she exited the room turning off the light. That day was never brought up again! However, the events of that night have never left my heart.

As I got older, I ended up with men who I knew weren't treating me the best, but I did not want to let them go. I was afraid. You may ask, "Afraid of what?" Afraid this was going to be as good as it got for me! After men would hit me—no, beat the hell out of me— they would tell me, "I love you very much. You know how mad I get. I didn't mean to do it. I will never, ever, ever do it again." I chose to foolishly believe them.

I honestly thought I could change the men I was in relationship with into the person I really believed that they could be. Surely I thought I could make them into the men I needed and wanted them to be exclusively for me. However, I really didn't know at all what or who I needed them to be. I often wonder would my life be different if my dad had shown me the love and affection I needed and desired. Would it have made an impact on the kind of men I allowed in my life? After all I've been through, I can now say that my dad is still my dad and I love him for who he is just the same.

What Childhood?

Another important and destructive factor in my life occurred between the ages of eight and twelve when I was repeatedly molested. I experienced some vile and disgusting acts. These acts were forced upon me by friends of my family. They were grownups, people that my family and I trusted. Some of the nastiest things that you can think of happening to a child happened to me. Grown men had sex with me, used their fingers to penetrate my vagina, ejaculated on my chest rather than completing their disgusting act inside of me. I did not know that they were intentionally trying to prevent impregnating me — a minor. They tongue kissed me and sucked on the knots on my chest. One of them even made me grab his penis to help him masturbate.

After all of those disgusting and violating acts were over, often times these molesters would shower me with gifts or compliments which satisfied me at the time and lead me to believe that what happened to me was okay and sometimes even consensual. You know the kind of compliments that every little girl needs, the "Oh, you're so good," "I love you," and "You're so pretty" compliments. Because of their unsolicited and unwelcome sick behavior, I suffered much confusion concerning relationships, emotions, and sex. My mentality concerning men was warped. I thought that if I gave them me, my body, and my emotions, maybe then, they would give me anything that I wanted including all the compliments and attention that are experienced in a committed relationship.

Those memories added more names to the list. Names that were unfairly connected to me through abuse and deception but they were nonetheless names God had told me to write down. The process burned a mixture of sorrow and anger in my chest. Through prayer and after several days, I began to understand that the more I gave my body and emotions, the more I was wooed into a false sense of confidence in these relationships, in the men, and in myself. I had acquired a bogus sense of comfort, mistaken perception of joy, and a deceptive impression of being loved. In essence, I learned how to be a whore in the flesh and in the spirit. In each of those relationships, I was not always praying like I should. I was not always studying the Word or getting to know God like I should. I was running around serving, giving my entire being. I hadn't yet realized that what I was looking for could only be found in the security of a relationship rooted in Jesus Christ.

The Terrible Teens

As a result of the molestation, by the time I became a teenager I willingly did some awful things. At fourteen, I became involved with an older teenage boy who performed oral sex on me on a regular basis. I was taught how to French kiss by a forty-two-year old man who also enjoyed touching me. When I was fifteen, I had become so confused that I had a sexual encounter with a nineteen-year-old female who was a lesbian. At the time, the rationale I felt in my heart of hearts was that I had to become perfect in all acts of the flesh and lust. It was the driving force for me to get whatever I wanted while giving others what they wanted. However, the truth was I had no real idea what I wanted.

I felt that I had nothing else to offer anyone except my body. I wasn't light skinned, as it seemed most men preferred, and I wasn't pretty or even shapely. So I lived in a man's hidden world which usually was his bed. I never felt pretty, even on my best days. I always felt that I lacked some physical beauty that would make men treat me special. I wasn't sure what it was, but I knew that I wasn't whole. Was it the bags under my eyes, my small chest, or my big nose? Oh, he must be treating me this way because I'm as dark as night, I often convinced myself.

While I thought through that memory, I tried to stop the flow of thoughts for a moment. I tried focusing on my family by cooking dinner, helping my daughter with her homework, cleaning the house. I wanted to do anything to clear my mind of the past God was placing before me. I was praying that this process would be deliverance and it would bring me closer to God. I couldn't bear continuing on and on down memory lane without His hand guiding me. When I returned to my designated prayer time in this consecration, God met me with more memories as if I had only pressed pause in the story. He reminded me of a time when my God-sister drove me to a very popular hangout in the city.

While there I saw my first boyfriend whom I dated when I was sixteen. He came over to the car and we started talking, basically about nothing and before I knew it my current boyfriend was at the car. He began to frantically beat on the car window asking us what was going on. He looked at my ex-boyfriend and asked him why was he all in my face, and then added you must be sleeping with her. They were arguing back and forth. A fight was waiting to happen.

My boyfriend looked at me and shouted, "Get your *** to the house now!" After my boyfriend and my ex-boyfriend finished their argument, one saying what he was going to do to me and the other saying, "You ain't gone do ****!" I told my ex I would be ok, but I knew I had better go! Out of fear, I did exactly what he said. I dropped off my God-sister and went straight home. As I pulled up in the yard, he was pulling up directly behind me. We got out of our cars and walked towards each other. Before I could say a word; he threw a closed fist punch that landed on my eye causing me to fall to the ground. Once on the ground he proceeded to kick me in my face, back, head, and stomach, dragging me by my hair with every blow. When he was done, he went back to his car where his friend sat watching and waiting. When he was done, he left me there on the ground. My neighbors watched me. Yes, they watched as I attempted to stand, but my knees kept giving out on me, and I would fall back to the ground. So I dragged myself to my back door and went inside the house.

I made it to the bathroom and sat on the toilet seat. I wasn't crying because I was more in shock than anything else. I was wondering why I couldn't see. I had not seen my face yet, but when I noticed the blood on my clothes and hands and felt it dripping from my face, I decided to look in the mirror. And that's when I started crying. My face was a horrible mess, swollen eye, knots on my forehead, swollen jaw, busted lips. I didn't even recognize myself!

How could my sweet, drug dealing, loving, weed smoking, sexy, daddy to seven babies, cute, cheating boyfriend do this to me? At the time I didn't recognize this as domestic violence. All I know is that when I looked in the mirror, reality hit. It was not until I saw myself that I realized "oh my God, he just beat me unrecognizable". The mirror told the true story. I saw a helpless, defenseless naïve little girl who was out of her league, wondering in an area that she knew not.

That night my mom was at work. After surviving this brutal beating, my boyfriend began to swear that he was scared of my mother. Afraid of what she might do to him if we were still there when she got home and saw what he had done to me. What he really meant was if she called the police on him, he was sure to go to jail. So, he packed me a few things while I sat on my bed and cried—holding both my jaw and my eye. We would go to the hotel, a place where we did not have to see my mother at least until the next day.

Once at the hotel, he pampered me, putting ice on my swollen and cut eye and ran my bath water. Then, after reassuring me it would never happen again, we "made" sex. Yes, I said we made sex because love does not leave you with a swollen eye, swollen jaw, busted lips, and blood clots in your eyes.

I had the worst headache from him dragging me by my hair as I fell from the beating he had rendered upon me in the street. Yes, I was beaten in the street as onlookers watched and refused to get involved. You would think that after having no one come to my rescue or even call the police that I would be mad at everyone who witnessed such an act. But I wasn't! I was, however, ashamed and embarrassed that my boyfriend was beating me. I felt scared and confused about what I had done to deserve such a beating from someone, who had just the night before, professed his love for me as he made "sex" to me so gently. I was angry with myself for whatever I had done and even thought, as I dragged myself up the stairs to my back door. Maybe this is from something I did to someone else, something I sowed and now I'm reaping.

This relationship continued with much of the same pattern until one day, we were arguing, and I watched his face turn beat red right before my eyes. He was overcome with anger and he raised his fist at me and said, "I ought to beat the **** out of you!" At that moment I had a glimpse into my future. I saw this man beating me, belittling me, and torturing me for the rest of my life. And it was at that very moment that I said to him, "If you do, it will be your last time! I am tired of this!" He left my home that day and I didn't see him again till many years later!

While these experiences were not pleasant, I thank God I survived! Even in my sin, He still protected me and had a purpose for my life— purpose established before the foundation of the world. His love was unsearchable and it has not changed even today. At that time, I did not know anything about how to love.

About five years later, I was just beginning to learn and understand more about the Lord God and myself when I was introduced to these scriptures:

> *If I speak in the tongues of men and of angels, but have not love, I am a noisy gong or a clanging cymbal. And if I have prophetic powers and understand all mysteries and all knowledge, and if I have all faith, so as to remove mountains, but have not love, I am nothing. If I give away all I have, and if I deliver up my body to be burned, but have not love, I gain nothing. Love is patient and kind; love does not envy or boast; it is not arrogant or rude. It does not insist on its own way; it is not irritable or resentful; it does not rejoice at wrongdoing, but rejoices with the truth. Love bears all things, believes all things, hopes all things, and endures all things. Love never ends. "*
>
> 1 Corinthians 13:1-8, NIV

> *"So now faith, hope, and love abide, these three; but the greatest of these is love."*
>
> 1 Corinthians 13:13, NIV

The man who inflicted such a horrible beating on me was shot in the back after an altercation with another young man. When I received the news, I called him at the hospital to tell him that God loved him and that I had forgiven him for everything that he had done to me. He said, "Shaun, I always thought you hated me after the things I had done and said to you." I responded by saying, "I never stopped caring about you, and no matter what you did to me, I would never have wished such harm on anyone."

Years later, my friend called to tell me that he had died from stomach cancer and had left at least eight children behind. I got off the phone crying, not rejoicing. I cried out, "Lord, please tell me that he had surrendered his life to you before he was taken away."

Even after this relationship, I continued on for many years allowing this pattern of sexual, physical, verbal, and emotional abuse to rule my life. I had not figured out yet who I was to or in the Lord God completely. I went from one relationship to another, carrying bags of anger, hurt, insecurities, depression, and low self-esteem. I realize now that hurting people hurt other people. I was one of those hurting people hurting others. In my own hurt, I realized that I affected the lives of those closest to me.

I had many outbursts of anger. I wanted those around me to hurt and feel what I felt because no one bothered to ask me what was going on. It did not seem as though anyone really cared. If someone had asked what was going on with me, I would have had no problem telling them. All I knew is that I wanted to be happy and I made my happiness other people's responsibility. This attitude is known as co-dependency, which is another book all in itself.

Then, I had my first consensual sexual experience with my boyfriend. He was twenty-two years old and, in my mind, he was by far the best thing that had ever happened to me. We dated for more than a year. He was a hard-working young man, and not a "self-employed" drug dealer. While with him, I was exposed to a different lifestyle, one much calmer and more stable than anything I had ever experienced. He never focused on sex, but in my ignorance, sex was what I thought a relationship was made of so that's what I focused on. I was definitely the aggressor. As time passed, I began to talk myself into believing that he was too conservative for me.

When I broke off this relationship, another destructive phase of my life began. By the eleventh and twelfth grades, I was even more of a mess. At first, I began skipping certain classes, and gradually started skipping school all together. I would meet up at friends' houses to smoke weed, go to the mall, and of course to have sex. During this time, my parents separated which eventually led to divorce. I chose to live with my mom who worked twelve- to fourteen-hour days. She was totally oblivious to the extent of my reckless behavior. I eventually dropped out of school, and my life continued to spiral out of control.

I saw other girls dating drug dealers and I thought that was what I also wanted. This was so attractive to me because the one thing I noticed in the drug game was that it didn't matter so much about your looks. Your clothes, jewelry, money, and cars would make you or break you in the streets. With any of those things, you could look like a booger bear and have women or men lined up down the street and around the corner waiting for you. In my mind, it was easier to dress up the outer me and gain some type of acceptance than to reveal that I was a little girl, hurting on the inside, just wanting to be seen for myself. I was lost in a grown-up body, doing grown-up things just wanting to be loved, accepted, and nurtured . (This holds true for many teenagers today.)

Please Don't Leave Me Alone!

I've watched countless television programs where many young women talked about how they were promiscuous because they had low self-esteem. The women would admit that they did not feel pretty and the guys would re-affirm them by confessing their love.I used to be one of those young women and I recognized that the issue is deeper than having low self-esteem, wishing to be pretty, and desiring to feel loved in the natural. The issue is spiritual.

I have had it said to me before, "Those kids don't want to hear that stuff, especially if they don't ask!" To that I say, "WHAT, are you serious?" When I was younger, I did not ask because I did not have enough sense to ask. And at times, adults can seem like the enemy, especially when they don't share their truths. I can remember when I was walking around with pink hair, blue finger nails, panties on (because they sure did not look like the shorts they were supposed to be), and gold teeth, people would make assumptions. They would say things like, "Child, she's just hot. She's too far gone to help Let her keep on, she'll see." Well, all of that may have been true to the on-looker, but God searches the heart and so should we.

During that time of my life, my body language, dress, and attitude suggested that I simply wanted to be left alone. However, just like some of our kids today, I really wanted some caring adult to touch me on the shoulder and lovingly say, "What in the world are you doing?" I thank God for the people in my life who saw the best in me when everyone around me chose to see the worst in me. I appreciate God for the prayers of the righteous that sustained my life. I am so grateful to God for the few who said, "Yes, you are a mess now. You are torn-up from the floor up. You are headstrong and hard-headed, but God!"

I truly thank God for the few people who continued to pour out God's love upon me. Even when I was drinking, getting high, rebellious, and having sex not only like it was going out of style, but like it was the only style. They saw what I didn't see: the fact that there was a hope for my future and that it would not be cut off! Even when I continued in my sin, God knew my end from the beginning.

Love or Lust? There is a Difference

I Gave Up Many Things For What I Thought Was Love – My Peace, My Anointing, and My Freedom.

As a young woman, I was in so much lust with one particular young man that I was doing, and willing to do, anything for him all because he said he loved me. I met this young man while walking to the local store in my neighborhood. He was cute, charming, and a bona fide thug. Before I knew it, I was being wined and dined. I was eating at nice restaurants not fast food drive-ups. I was staying at some of the ritziest hotels for weeks at a time. In my mind, I was living the dream life. This young man gave mea lot of money to do with as I pleased. Sometimes he would give me hundreds of dollars easily. But I quickly learned that life isn't fair or free.

As the relationship continued, I started trafficking drugs from one state to another for my boyfriend. He promised me that one day we would get married and live happily ever after. In between the cussing, beatings, and other abusive moments, I really believed that somewhere down the road, we would get married because we loved each other. Nothing changed my mind. Not even when his baby's momma threw a brick through the kitchen window of my home hoping he was home with me when he was not. Yet, I continued the relationship with him. He could have been with any other woman that night, and I still continued the relationship with him.

One day, his baby's momma demanded that he chose between me or her and his response was "both of you need to quit the drama because neither of you are going anywhere." When it was over, she left crying and he and I drove back to our hotel room, together. Was I ignorant, stupid or crazy? The bottom line is that I thought I was in love.

As I reflected back, God led me to the first time I actually trafficked illegal drugs for this man. I was ignorant and I would do anything for love and attention! One day, we headed out of town and the sheriff's department stopped the bus we were on. Stepping onto the bus were three deputy sheriff's being charming, but ready to make a bust at the same time. One sheriff stopped in front, one stopped midway and the other went straight to the back. As they approached us, T was so nervous, while I was too stupid to understand the severity of what was going on around me.

We just happened to be sitting smack dab in the middle of the bus. The sheriff looked at us and asked if we would mind if he searched our bags. I agreed and I pointed overhead to the bag that was ours. He began with small talk, asking, "You two married?"

"No," I said.

"Where you all going?" he said.

"Oh, we're headed out of town to meet with family, and I'm going to introduce my boyfriend to them for the first time!"

He started to smile and said, "Man, you ready for that?" My boyfriend just smiled. Now the whole time the officer is talking and searching I had no fear because I was carrying the drugs, covered by socks and a pair of boots.

Fortunately, the sheriff sent the bus along its way after checking underneath the bus. Instead, the first thing I said to T was, "I told you I got this," when the bus started moving again. Well, that encounter made my boyfriend so nervous that he swore I would never carry anymore drugs on me again. He decided that I would stick to cutting and bagging the drugs only. Looking back on that decision, what kind of pronouncement was that? But, at the time, it did not matter; I just wanted to be in T's presence.

Once back home from what we called a successful run, we suited up to go out again. Holding true to his word, I carried no drugs. T paid one of his good friends to go with us and carry all things illegal in a duffle bag. We were riding the city bus, going along good until we get stopped AGAIN in the same area by the same sheriff's department. I thought we would will be okay. They didn't do much the last time, in fact, they were on and off the buses in no time. But they shocked everyone on bus when they got on with K-9s. Fear overtook me, not for myself but for what was going to happen to T's friend.

Sitting across from us and one row ahead, we could see him clearly with the bag placed on the floor between his feet. When they started inching their way to the back, we were all stiff. One of the oversized German Sheppards went into a frenzy, barking at the black traveling bag under his seat. Deputy Sheriffs surrounded him took the bag and politely asked him if he would get off the bus. He did. I think the next time I saw him was at least five years later when he got out of prison. You would think, okay, end of business, right? Not so! T simply decided, "No more buses," and started driving after that! I get chills every time I think of that day.

I didn't even know to say, "Thank you, God for covering me!" I never even acknowledged Him. Now, I pause and realize that God sent ministering angels to a worthless, naïve person like me, because He saw more in me, while I was in my sin than I saw in myself on my best days which were few and far between.

Later that same year, T went to make a drug deal without me (by God's grace). He ended up selling drugs to some undercover DEA agents and spent the next eight years in prison. The whole situation affected everybody who was connected to us in some way. Once T was arrested, my aunt who often allowed us to stay with her when we were on her side of town, completely unaware of what we were doing, immediately wanted to help my boyfriend. So, she offered to put her house up for him as collateral to help. What a bad decision that was in every way you look at it. I, for one, didn't even have enough sense to tell her not to give up the home she'd lived in for more than twenty-five years. I didn't look at how this would affect an already strained relationship with my family. I only knew it was a way to get him out of jail!

Sure enough, he was released from jail on bond. He swore to me that he was done with that lifestyle and that he just wanted to get away for a little while to think. He promised me that he would be back in time for his upcoming court charges of drug trafficking and more. Why did I believe that?

The court date came and went. Threats from the bondsmen started coming concerning my aunt's home. The bondsmen found their way to my front door. They wanted my boyfriend at all costs.

I explained to them I had not seen him in at least three days. Honestly, even if I would have known where he was, I would not have told them.

They asked me to take them to a couple of places where I thought he might be. I really did not know where he was staying, but I went with them anyway. Needless to say, we did not find him. The next morning, my boyfriend called me saying, "Baby, don't start crying, because if you do, I'm going to hang up on you." I said, "What's wrong?" He said, "I am on my way to prison; I awoke to guns and pistols in my face this morning." Yes, the bondsmen had found him. One of his family members had turned him in. I was devastated! I started crying and screaming. He said, "Baby, I need you to stop crying or I am going to hang up the phone." Suddenly, I heard a dial tone. It was three months before he called again.

I am encouraged to say that my aunt is still in her home; however, for many years I walked in guilt and condemnation because of the position I put her in and what it could have cost her. I take full responsibility! I have asked my aunt to forgive my foolish, immature, and selfish action, and she said, "There's nothing to forgive, Baby. I love you, Sugar."I am thankful to my auntie for forgiving me. If the truth be told, that whole ordeal shook me straight! No, not straight, as in changing my behavior for the better, but "straight" as in exploring "safer" acts of sin. Instead o dealing drugs, I got more into drinking, smoking weed, and clubbing, and let's not forget that demon that sat on my back longer, heavier, and bigger than any other: fornication.

Reflecting on the Past

Past situations, abuse, and experiences which had nothing to do with him had become attached to me. I was damaged emotionally and did not know what it meant to be in a real loving relationship. This man knew that there had been many past hurts in my life and said that he would love me no matter what. Instead of embracing someone who knew how foolish I could be and understood that I had some growing up to do, I rejected him. Someone willing to walk me through it all, and still choose to love me, I rejected him. I was damaged goods. And in my mind, I didn't know if any man, or even I for that matter, would ever deem me worth anything but sex.

Don't Pass the Buck

For years, I lived and walked in that false way of thinking. One day I was singing the song, "This joy that I have, the world didn't give it, and the world cannot take it away." When I finished singing that song, I asked myself this question, "How do you know if you have ever had joy?" As I pondered this question, I asked God to reveal an answer to me. And this is the scripture, He led me to:

David spoke about him. He said, 'I know that the Lord is always with me. He is at my right hand. I will always be secure. So my heart is glad. Joy is on my tongue. My body also will be full of hope. You will not leave me in the grave. You will not let Your Holy One rot away. You always show me the path that leads to life. You will fill me with joy when I am with You.

Acts 2:25-28, NIRV

David says, "YOU, Lord, fill me with joy when I am with You and in Your presence." True joy comes from worshiping, spending time and being filled with Him! I cannot thank God enough for finally being in a place now where I am opening myself up to learn more about Him and myself. This helps me to understand my mother and father better. It would be so easy to blame them for my wrong decisions, hurts, and pains. While I know all parents have some form of responsibility when it comes to the upbringing of their children, in this season of mirrors and self reflection, I pass the buck to no one.

"Each one should test his own actions. Then he can take pride in himself, without comparing himself to somebody else, for each one should carry his own load."

Galatians 6: 4-5, NIV

It's Not Over until God Says It's Over!

One day, about mid-way into this season on mirrors, I remember a neighbor who I grew up with. She was so sweet, quiet, and even a little shy. When she got pregnant one, two, three, and four times, I remember teasing her saying, "Girl, what are you doing?" Well, a few years and six children later she was dead. I cried for weeks asking God why her!

She had so much to live for, especially for her children. Her children were her life. The number one thing I think of when I think of her is how kind she was. To die at such a young age, twenty-five or so, I asked again, "Why not me, Lord? Why were You saving me? She and I lived a similar lifestyle. Why are you shielding me?"

I sat in my car with my notepad that had pages of names. "Lord. I have slept with more guys than she did, why wasn't it me?"

I had no children. My relationship with my family was non-existent and at that time I saw no real hope or future for my life. I would have traded my life so she could have been here with her children. And, I can recall hearing a still small voice, which I believed to be the voice of God saying, "It's not over for you, Boo, until I say it's over!"

I knew God or should I say knew of God. I was taught from a little girl attending church that God loved me however I never could comprehend the depth of His love for me. I did not fully understand or know God for myself until, many, many years later.

I was at a Bible study in the home of my friend Marilyn. We were studying this scripture:

Ask, and it shall be given you, seek and ye shall find; knock, and it shall be open unto you for every one that asketh receiveth and he that seeketh findeth; to him that knocketh it shall be open
Matthew 7:7-8 .

I took this scripture to heart and studied it like no other. It just seemed too simple but I tried Him by asking for divine revelation of scripture as I studied and read. I wanted clarity on the spirit of discernment that had been prophesied to me my whole life. I also wanted the gift of speaking in other tongues, and yes, God granted my requests.

Even then, I kept being as destructive as I could be. I drank, smoked blunts, and had sex as often as I liked. Eventually, I got pregnant. The father told me he had enough kids and did not want anymore. I was devastated. I thought, "Well, he does not want any more children, and I do not need or deserve the one I'm having."

So I found a clinic that performed abortions and scheduled to have one. On the day of my appointment, my boyfriend did not accompany me because he was out of town selling drugs. So, one of my friends went with me. At the time, it was seemingly the best decision to make, and it appeared to be easy the first time, because after it was all over, I distracted myself with weed, alcohol, and the lie that it was the best thing for everyone involved! However, truth be told, at that time I had no real thought or understanding of the severity of what I had done, not only to my body or my unborn child, but to my spirit overall.

After two more pregnancies, one that ended in another abortion and one that I miscarried, I still did not think about the toll that this was having on my body. I surely was not thinking about my spiritual walk because I had none at the time. This is why today it is so hard for me to see these teen babies around me making the same perilous choices. To not reach out to them about God's truth, is to me a sin in itself.

> *Do you not know that your body is a temple of the*
> *Holy Spirit, who is in you, whom you have received*
> *from God? You are not your own*
> *I Corinthians 6:19, NIV*

I remember, one night I was on the phone with a friend of mine, who is not only a powerhouse in Jesus, but has been able to combine her love for people and her ministry into one. She is a God-appointed nurse. As we were talking and sharing our love and passion for helping and encouraging young people, I gave her an analogy of how passionate I am that just blew her mind. I said to her: "Just imagine driving by and seeing an accident. Then, you stop and run over asking how you can help. You see the police, the ambulance, and several other people standing around. Near the injured, hurting person lay all the tools necessary to help them, but the crew that's there says it's not their call. So they just watch and wait. Now, when you look at all these people and determine that they are crazy, and something has to be done, you proceed to help but someone puts their hand across your chest saying, 'Just leave them there till the next person comes.' As you fight to get to them in order to help them, they die!"

That's how I feel when I see young people, especially young women, who are giving their bodies and emotions away to people who don't care anything about them. These young women are walking around with no real understanding of what they are doing to their bodies, emotions, and their futures. I am no one's savior, but the Word of God is soul saving, and it says:

> *All this is from God, who reconciled us to himself through Christ and gave us the ministry of reconciliation: that God was reconciling the world to*

himself in Christ, not counting people's sins against them. And he has committed to us the message of reconciliation.

2 Corinthians 5:18-19

Jazzy

One of God's Greatest Gifts

When I got pregnant with my daughter Jazzy, I was determined that I was going to have her no matter what the cost. I had come to a place in my life where I believed that God was telling me that there were no more outs for me. I realized that I had to start checking myself and that it's not the baby's fault when it comes to decisions about aborting a life. It was my unwise and selfish decision, no matter the reasoning. I had to first recognize what and why that seemed to be my first choice and then I had to change my thinking! And I did.

Deep inside I felt that I did not have a choice in if I would birth Jazzy. Although she was a product of my selfish and unwise choices, I knew in my heart that she was destined to be! Before getting pregnant with Jazmin, I was living a carefree, careless life. I was still not using condoms or any other form of protection with any of my partners. As a result of this behavior, I have wrestled with the guilt of not knowing who Jazmin's biological father is. I have always openly shared my life with my daughter: the good, the bad and the ugly. I have apologized and repented to my daughter for my behavior. I have also instilled in her what God truly designed our bodies to be used for and what not to be used for. I have also shared this next passage of scripture with her on several occasions, because I felt no other scripture could have said what I wanted to say better:

> *And don't you realize that if a man joins himself to a prostitute, he becomes one body with her? For the Scriptures say, 'The two are united into one.' But the person who is joined to the Lord is one spirit with Him. Run from sexual sin! No other sin so clearly affects the body as this one does. For sexual immorality is a sin against your own body. Don't you realize that your body is the temple of the Holy Spirit, who lives in you and was given to you by God? You do not belong to yourself, for God bought you with a high price. So you must honor God with your body.*
> *1 Corinthians 6:16-20, New Living Translation*

Since Jazmin is older now, we talk more about the man that could possibly be her father. This is one of the greatest tasks put on my plate, but one that I am motivated to achieve because of my daughter. When I look at Jazmin, I have no regrets at all about birthing her. Although, there are many nights when I have cried and grieved the murder of my aborted children due to my own ignorance.

Reapin' and a Sowin'
Sowin' and a Reapin'

During this consecration, I had to remind myself and praise God that today my life is so much different. I would oftentimes say this prayer.

Father, as I sit here in the sanctuary in your presence, I am thankful for being here. I came under attack this morning in my mind. A lie was told to me over and over again. What lie? The one that says I am not worthy. It asks why even go to church? You are such a failure. But God, I believe there is hope for me. You are my hope. Because of your love for me, I press toward the mark of a higher calling... Christ Jesus, I receive peace in my mind, my thoughts, and my heart. The way is already made for me. I don't know what it is, but I do know this: that you know, in fact, you are the way.

I come to you broken but still believing; damaged but not destroyed; confused but not cut off from Your grace; hurt but not hopeless. I thank You God for loving me in the midst of my madness. I know that You are not finished with me yet. You are a wonderful King, a Savior like none other. Your love, kindness, grace, mercy, will, pose for my life, and forgiveness endure. One psalmist with Shekinah Glory says,

Jesus, how He loves me I'll never know." Lord, I'll never know, but I am grateful that you do. In your name, Jesus, I pray.

Your Daughter

God has given me a heart to help keep young girls from going down the path of destruction I once headed down. One thing I always try to instill in teenagers is for them to take care of this earthen vessel we call a body. Guard it with your life, because it's the only one we have. When I began to speak these words, I was completely unaware of what was ahead for me.

However, as I sat with God during this time of consecration, I realize there were times that I knew better and I boldly chose to do differently. I think about how I did what I wanted to do with no thought of the consequences that would follow.

Once, one of the youth who I considered as my child, discovered she was pregnant and she reminded me of myself. She was so upset and so very scared. She was afraid to tell her father who was a pastor. I was able to share my personal testimony with her. I told her how there are consequences for everything that we do, good or bad. I spoke to her about what we must do is take responsibility for our part in order to go forward and leave with a greater since of knowledge than what we started with. I said everything I knew to say to comfort her and help her make sense of where she was now and what direction she needed to head towards for her future and the future of her unborn child. I was able to comfort and encourage her, not as one who had it all together, but as one who says I still do not know everything, but what I do know is this! God knows everything, and because He does, I have had to learn day by day to lean and depend upon His Word to keep me! Keep me through sexual sin, my mental diagnosis, low self esteem and so much more.

> *There is surely a future hope for you, and your hope will not be cut off.*
> *Proverbs 23:18, NIV*

During my many years of sexual sin, I was never concerned about the cost and how my body would pay the price many years later. I was sexually active and self-destructive; but, more than that, I was sexually active with no thought of protecting myself. I accepted that age old lie that "it feels better without one." It was a lie then and it is still a lie now. Unprotected sex is sure to bring one of two things: a sexually transmitted disease or pregnancy. I was experienced both!

I remember when the doctor first told me I had an STD, which had been given to me by my sexual partners who were also partnering sexually with other people. After the doctor administered a shot in the butt and prescribed a ten-day supply of antibiotics, I thought, "How in the world could this happen to me?" But in all honesty, how could it not? I was concerned about that temporary feeling and not the longterm consequences.

After such an awful experience you would think I would have stopped having sex or ran to the nearest store and purchased every condom available. However, once again, no such thought entered my mind. Instead, I continued having unprotected sex. I often look back and ask myself, "Why? What was I thinking?" But if the truth be told, I was not thinking. I was too busy feeling!

While speaking with a group of young ladies about some of the things that I had been through and how God's grace and mercy were the only things that kept me, I said, "When we give up our bodies to a man who is not our husband, we not only sin against God, but it is also like being a prostitute." One of the young ladies asked, "Why do you say that? A prostitute?"

I responded, "Yes, a prostitute because, when you look at it, you are saying, 'I'll give you this part of me if you'll love me, stay with me, or pay me!'"

Oftentimes, I think we stereotype a prostitute or hooker as some nasty woman who gives up her goods to anybody and everybody. We see a prostitute as some dirty drug addict, and that is not always the case. If we are not mindful of our bodies, we can find ourselves partaking in the same acts and motives without it being a professional part of our lives. We must remember that there is no big or little sin. Sin is sin. Whether we defile our vessels with one man or one hundred and one men, we have still sinned against God by abusing and misusing our precious bodies.

> *"Food for the stomach and the stomach for food—but God will destroy them both. The body is not meant for sexual immorality, but for the Lord, and the Lord for the body."*
>
> *I Corinthians 6:13*

My True Husband has Arrived —Says Me!

The revelation that really broke me was the God's disdain for adultery. During this consecration he reminded me of Mr. Handsome.

My Prince Charming! I can remember the first day I met him as if it was yesterday. It was a typical weekday morning. I started the day preparing for work and getting my Jazzy ready for school. The typical early morning rush. We finally got it together and hurried downstairs to the car. Before we got into the car I noticed, to my disappointment, I had a flat tire. I walked back up the stairs to call my job and notify them of the situation and to undress Jazzy as I had no other way of getting her to school. I decided that Jazzy and I would just stay home, get back in our beds, and relax. Shortly after getting comfortable and noticing that an hour or so had passed, I decided to walk next door to the rental office. When I walked in, my landlord was having a conversation with a strikingly tall, dark, and handsome man (6'3", 350lbs). I politely interrupted their conversation and asked if she knew of anyone who could help fix my flat tire. And of course, Mr. Handsome was kind enough to volunteer to assist me.

Happy that I would be receiving help to get my car back in commission, I led him to my car. As he proceeded to get the spare tire out of the trunk of my car, he saw my car tag which read, "GODB4ME". He looked at me and said, "Read that car tag!" I thought sarcastically, "Ooh, Lord, great… He is tall, dark and absolutely handsome, but can't read a lick. What in the world?" He repeated the tag inscription two more times; as if he could not believe someone would have such a tag on their license plate. He concentrated on my plate then started fixing the tire. He initiated about the Lord, ministry, and a lot of various subjects. When he was finally done fixing the flat tire, he said, "LeShaun, I would like to give you my number." I told him that I really appreciated his help, but calling him was out of the question. He responded, "If you are not led by God to call me, then don't call!" He placed the number in my hand and left.

Later that night after putting my princess to bed, I began to think about my tire being flat, and the fact that I went over to that rental office and happened to meet that young man there.

It was about 8:30 that evening when I dialed his number and he answered. Surprised to hear from me, we quickly engaged in a lively conversation.We talked about everything above and under the sun. It was a beautiful, wholesome, clean conversation filled with refreshing perspectives and ideas. It was so exciting and new to my soul—mind, will, and emotions. We shared our inner most hurts, failures and successes.

I talk to him about my feelings of having a mental illness and how it has affected my Christian walk. How I sometimes felt like the very last place I could go to vent all of my woes and concerns with being labelled was the church. And in our sharing he revealed to me that he was married, officially separated, and living apart for more than a year. We did not get off the phone until his alarm clock sounded to let him know that it was time to go to work at 6:30 in the morning!

During each of our conversations, I learned so much more about him. He was a minister, music director for the praise and worship team for his church, and fourteen years older than I was. All of these facts worked in his favor. From the first morning we got off that phone, we kept the regimen of having great conversations for hours, very long hours. Then one day, during one of our extended conversations, he dropped the big one on me.

He asked if I would let him cook dinner for me. I thought, *Oh, yes, Lord!* I was so excited and impressed, but I couldn't let him know it. I wanted to show him that I was mature and serious about my relationship with God so I responded, "Well, dinner sounds nice; however, may I bring one of friends and mentor?" He said, "LeShaun, you can bring the whole church. I just would like for you to be present."

Minister Mason, who keeps me in line in every area of my life, joined us for dinner and enjoyed a fabulous meal, one in which I did not have to assist at all. He wanted me just to feel welcomed. This man would not even allow me to wash dishes after we finished eating. It was just amazing! As we allowed our food to settle, he pulled out his keyboard and proceeded to play. We sang, laughed, and talked about the things that the Lord had brought us through. Two days after the dinner date, he gave me a key to his home.

"I'm giving you this key, not to move in, but to come over relax, eat or whatever, even when I'm not in," he said graciously.

As time progressed, I would go and cleanup for him. Sometimes I would bring my little one with me other times she would be with my God-mother Mother Givhan or with my sister Youlunda. One time, while my daughter was at school, I ironed every piece of clothing in his closet. When he got home from church, he called me at home in utter excitement, "Baby, you ironed my clothes!" Then, corrected himself, "I'm sorry, I meant to say, LeShaun, you ironed all of my clothes." He was so happy, and I had a desire to always make him happy. But, we all know that there is always something lurking to try to shatter your happiness. So part of me waited to see what that something would be to shatter this relationship for me.

One night later, Jazzy experienced a very high fever and diarrhea. All she could do was cry. I called Mr. Handsome to tell him what was happening and he asked if he could bring Gatorade and other things that might get rid of the fever and pain. Being that it was a nearly midnight and I did not want to take Jazzy out in that condition, I told him that I would be grateful if he did.

When he arrived, Jazzy was on the toilet still experiencing flu and cold like symptoms. He came with everything he thought could help. About 1:30 the next morning, Jazzy's fever had gone down quite a bit and the diarrhea had completely stopped. My baby finally went to sleep two hours later. As I continued to hold her in my arms for the remainder of the morning, he and I sat talking on the couch in the living room.

We cracked jokes and laughed, especially once I knew Jazzy was going to be okay. Before, we knew it, dawn had rolled around and he got up to go home so that he could get ready for work. For some reason, through that whole ordeal, I felt that God was not only showing me how much Mr. Handsome loved me, but He was also showing me that I was worthy of being loved. Loved by someone who did not abuse my mind, body, or spirit, and had remained a Godly gentleman at all costs.

God is a God of His Word!

One Sunday night in February, Jazzy and I met Mr. Handsome at his house for dinner. He gave us each a bouquet of beautiful roses and separate cards. I believe this was on February nineteenth, to be exact. As we sat on the couch watching one of those children's channels, which was shear entertainment for Jazzy, he pulled me close to him. I felt his warm embrace and heard his comforting words as he said, "LeShaun, you know that I love you."

I replied, "Yes, I do."

"I need you to know something. If I were to die today, God has done just what He said that He was going to do in my life."

I could not help but say, "What? Why are you talking like that? I don't want to hear that." In spite of my plea to stop talking nonsense, he continued to make his point by speaking in a low, loving tone. "I need you to listen. God promised me that for all of the hurt and pain I have had to endure over these last two years, He was going to restore unto me double. Double peace, double joy, double love, double confidence, just double blessings in every area. And, I want you to know that He has paid me double through my relationship with you and Jazzy. So if I die tomorrow, please know that God is a God of His Word and He's done just what He said He would do in my life."

The following night, I went by his home after work to cook enough spaghetti for him to eat for a few days. As I arrived, he was preparing to leave. The church bus was picking him up to play at a revival in another city. When I was done cooking, I left his home and remember looking at his car in the nearby parking space, thinking *What kind of parking is that?* He had backed into the spot leaving both front tires turned so far to the right that they looked stuck almost. I just laughed and went on my way. When he returned home from the revival, about twelve thirty the next morning, he called with such joy in his heart. He talked about how God "showed out," blessing people in a way that they could not have imagined. Because he was so exhausted from his day we decided to end the conversation early.

A Day to Remember

On the following Tuesday, I woke up super happy just like I had since the first night Mr. Handsome and I talked! When I finished getting Jazzy and myself ready for our day, out the door we went. As soon as I got to work, I realized that I had not received my morning call from him. I knew that his work kept him busy so I did not sweat it at first. However, by noon, I still had not gotten a phone call from him and it was at that point that I began to worry. I called him numerous times, but he was not answering his cell phone. I remembered he had a two o'clock doctor's appointment that he could not miss. Up until this point, I had never called his job, because I knew he worked mostly in the field. This time was a different circumstance, and I felt it warranted a phone call.

After taking a deep breath, I picked up the phone and I dialed the number to his job I trembled as the phone rang. Each ring seemed as though it was the longest one I had ever heard, and then the voice of the young female receptionist broke through the silence. Swallowing to keep from crying in the phone, I calmly asked her if he had come in to work that day. "Is this LeShaun?" She asked although I'd never met her.

I said, "Yes this is."

"No ma'am, we've not seen or heard from him today and that's just not like…" Before she could finish her sentence, I had dropped the phone, got up from my desk, grabbed my purse and keys, and ran to my car. I was speeding down the highway before I could take my next breath. I did not clock out, I did not inform anyone on my job that I was leaving, I was just out.

As I drove, I began to pray. "God, please just let him be home ignoring my calls." Even though that was not his character. I continued to pray, "Lord, just let his phone be broke. Just please let him be ok!" Grasping for any hope of peace, I then began to remember how I had seen his car the night before and I began to giggle at the memory of the way he had parked his car. It was a strange way to leave a car. After I turned the corner, I noticed his car was parked in the exact same way and in the very same space it had been the night before. My worst fears began to flood my mind, because I knew then that something was terribly wrong.. Visibly shaken and nervous, I walked up to the door and I used the key he had given me. The door wouldn't open because the chain latch was still in place. I anxiously called his name through the small space in the door; there was no response. I did this for several minutes, calling his name louder and louder as my heart beat harder and harder. I didn't know what else to do being that I could not get in. My mind led me to run and find the property maintenance person.

As soon as I located her, I frantically explained to her what was going on, and she said, "Let me grab my bolt cutters." When we arrived back, he still had not opened the door. So, she cut the chain. Normally, when I entered his home, I would go straight to the kitchen or the living room on the first floor. But this time, I ran straight upstairs screaming for him.

When I got upstairs, I turned to go in his room he was laying on the floor in his underwear. I rushed over and laid next to him crying hysterically, asking him what was wrong. There was no response. I tried to turn him over, but I was unable to. Then, I noticed he had released his bowels in his underwear and I began to scream louder.

The maintenance person came running up stairs. When she saw him on the floor, she said, "Oh my God, please move, get off of him!" But I couldn't. She grabbed the phone and called 9-1-1 for help. For the next few minutes, which felt like a few hours, I gently caressed his head, I kissed him, and I laid on his stiff body begging him desperately to please talk to me, "Please don't do this; please don't leave me!"

Finally, the ambulance arrived. Three uniformed men rushed into his home and surrounded us. I looked up, impulsively asking them to please help me. As they looked him over and assessed his vitals, one of them looked at me and said, "Ma'am, I'm sorry, he is dead. At this point there is nothing we can do to save him. We're sorry."

I started screaming and crying as they lifted me off of him. I just couldn't let him go. As I held on to him, they tried to free him from my grip. I began to plead, "Are you all even going to try to resuscitate him at all?" One of the paramedics responded, "I hear you, Ma'am, but he's gone. There is nothing we can do for him now."

I have often said that when they lifted and pulled me up from his lifeless body, my spirit laid there and never got up. For the next several months, I was depressed in a way I had never experienced before. In my heart, I felt his life was cut off too soon and that we were both cheated. I longed all my life to be able to be with someone who understood me, someone who understood my struggle and pain.

I was angry with God yes, angry with God! I didn't go to church. I didn't pray. All I did was cry, sit, stare at his obituary, and cry even more. I questioned why I had to find him? Why couldn't I have just gotten the call of his passing from someone else?

Mother Givhan, my mentor, and friend, would come over and attempt to talk to me. Even though I was unreceptive to any prayer, advice, word, or anything, she would still pray over me! Weeks turned into months of this same defiant rebellious behavior, and it was only the grace of God that kept me safe during this season. As I think back to one night in particular, these women of God came to my home to pray for me and to make sure I was doing well. Honestly, I was in no mood to be prayed for. Yes, I said it, and at the time, I meant it. I wanted to sit in self-pity and be alone. I wanted to cry and weep, "Woe is me!"

In the midst of all of these feelings and emotions, Mother Givhan and Prophetess Perry prayed for me. By the end of that visit, the Lord led Mother Givhan to give me a scripture from the book of Revelation which was given to the church of Ephesus. But, there was a relevant word in it just for me.

> *To the angel of the church in Ephesus write: 'These are the words of him who holds the seven stars in his right hand and walks among the seven golden lampstands. I know Your deeds, Your hard work, and Your perseverance. I know that You cannot tolerate wicked people, that You have tested those who claim to be apostles but am not, and have found them false. You have persevered and have endured hardships for*

my name, and have not grown weary. Yet, I hold this against you: You have forsaken the love you had at first. Consider how far you have fallen! Repent and do the things you did at first. If you do not repent, I will come to you and remove your lampstand from its place.

Revelation 2: 1-5, NIV

After she finished reading, she looked me right in the eye and said, "Now you meditate on this!" In her elderly way, she was saying, "You can't get so low that you don't want to hear a Word fromGod, work in the ministry or even pray. I know you are hurting and are in pain, I know you thought things were going to be different in this situation, but the truth is it didn't happen that way!"

At that time, I did not care to hear anything she was saying, I chose to sit in and not walk through the window of mourning that we are graced to receive. In Ecclesiastes 3:4, the Bible is clear that there's "a time to weep and a time to laugh, a time to mourn and a time to dance," which made me know that it was okay for me to mourn, but not to waddle in it; just as the Lord told Joshua:

After the death of Moses the servant of the Lord, the Lord said to Joshua son of Nun, Moses' aide: 2 "Moses my servant is dead. Now then, you and all these people, get ready to cross the Jordan River into

*the land I am about to give to them—to the Israelites.I
will give you every place where you set your foot, as I
promised Moses. Your territory will extend from the
desert to Lebanon, and from the great river, the
Euphrates—all the Hittite country—to the Great Sea
on the west. No one will be able to stand up against
you all the days of your life. As I was with Moses, so I
will be with you; I will never leave you nor forsake
you.*

Joshua 1:1-5, NIV

God was simply telling Joshua, "Okay, I know that Moses is gone,
but there is still work to be done so let's get it together." Well, of
course at the time, I did not get any of that and my response to it
was out of order and defiant. And that's when she said ,"You are
mourning the loss of a man you were deeming to one day be your
husband, but God is not going to give you somebody else's
husband to fulfill a promise to you. So, if you want to sit here like
this you can, but we will not be a part of it." As she and the
Prophetess were leaving she looked back at me and said,
"LeShaun, repent and do not forget your first love!"

Yes, he was married! Separated from his wife for more than a year
at the time we met, but married just the same. And, as far as God
was concerned, that marriage covenant between him and his wife
still stood! God later spoke to me and said, "LeShaun, I used you
to restore a broken man. I never intended for you to marry him;

but I intended for you to encourage, build, befriend and uplift him. I already knew what the end of that situation was going to be according to ME and My will! I wanted to teach you that you can have a man in your life whose only mission is to serve me and while serving me, show you the innocence of MY love!"

I went out of my way to justify why I felt my behavior was justifiable. One of my excuses was, "Oh, they're separated; they are not in the same house or even the same bed, so how could it be adultery?" I **used** ignorance as a right to willfully sin against God. I would say to myself, "Oh, I really did not know that applied to this situation." However, the covenant that was made between God, that man, and that woman, extended past them being in the same house. They were spiritually connected by God and by the law! What happens when you do know better and your excuses have been exhausted?

I found myself in a relationship with a man that I knew was married. According to him, he was unhappily married, but nevertheless he was still married! Unlike my previous relationship, in which the couple was already separated when I came into the picture, this man was still living with his wife. I made a conscious decision to fornicate with a man who by no means ever intended to leave his wife, no matter how miserable he claimed he was. If the truth be told, it was a spirit of lust, plain and simple. We did what we wanted to do because we wanted to. I remember many years ago my Bishop at the time would say, "Life is choice driven," and that held true then, and it still holds true today.

This consecration was turning more and more into the hardest forty days of my life! In the midst of this, God reminded me how one night while I was crying out to the Lord about my life and still questioning why? I was walking in the house Why me, and why so much pain? I told the Lord, "You didn't have to take him!" And at that moment, it felt like my whole house began to shake and I clearly heard the Lord say, "He belongs to me, who are you to contend with what I did and why I did it? I am God, and I made a promise to him and I used you to fulfill that promise. You should feel honored, not dishonored. I chose you to meet him, encourage him, and build him. I am a just God and there is nothing that happens to you or through you that I don't allow. Get over it!"

I repented and asked God to please forgive me, and guess what? He did, right at that very moment. Eventually, I did get over my selfish thinking. Who besides God loves us more? No one! To sacrifice His only begotten Son to save a filthy wretch like me, knowing even before I fall that I would be angry with him, giving into despair, hurt, and depression. HIS grace and mercy are sufficient for you and me!

And He has said to me, 'My grace is sufficient for you, for power is perfected in weakness.' Most gladly, therefore, I will rather boast about my weaknesses, so that the power of Christ may dwell in me.

II Corinthians 12:9

Why Does It Hurt So Bad

After losing Mr. Handsome, my life continued to be riddled with circumstances that would seemingly drive my mind and heart to some of the darkest places. I continued to live, or should I say, survive through up and down mood swings and many other emotional battles. My bouts of depression and suicidal thoughts were becoming deeper and darker. Suicide, I thought at the time, was a means to an end. I was so focused on the grief, pain of rejection, being misunderstood, and feelings of unworthiness. I believed that it would be easier on everyone around me if I simply were not here.

It was ALL a lie. Some days, I would just sleep all day. I would stay in the bed, in the dark, not even getting up to bathe. Suicidal thoughts invaded my mind. The only reason I did not commit suicide was because of Jazzy. I did not want her to find me. At one point, I'd tell myself she would be better off without me, then I'd struggle and push those thoughts back, believing she would be worse off without me. The grief around Mr. Handsome's death escalated thoughts and emotions that I'd struggled with year after year since childhood.

There was such a strong cry down within the depths of my soul of why me. Why do I have to struggle with this burden? My highs would be extremely high and my lows devastatingly low. I really wanted to understand what was going on with me. I knew I had accepted Jesus, but I could not figure out why I felt so bad. Why was the pain so deep? Why could I not get past the excruciating hurt and disappointments I felt?

After much prayer, I decided to go to the doctor. Following several evaluations, he gave me the diagnosis of bipolar disorder: depression and mania symptoms along with anxiety and panics attacks. Although that was not the news I expected to hear, I finally felt I had an answer to why I felt the way I did. Even though , I did not have the cure.

For years, I continued to wrestle with the demon of depression. Feeling more helpless and hopeless, and too weak to fight and carry this burden on my own, I decided to go seek professional help again. Upon additional evaluation, the doctor prescribed different medications for my diagnosis. I finally agreed to take the medications as prescribed in hopes that it would help me.

I was on and off at least seven different medications that did not work for me. After years of self-medicating with drugs, alcohol, and sex, and trying to figure out why I lived the way I did. Why could I not control my sporadic behavior? How could depression hit me in such a way that life seemed hopeless?

At times I would just stop taking the meds because I was told "If you're saved for real, you should not be taking anti-depressants like the world does." People would often tell me, "You might need to check your walk and see if you're saved!" Comments like these came from various people. I even heard similar remarks come from ministers during their sermons. I often felt that those kinds of comments came from people who did not understand, or even attempt to understand other people's struggles. My struggle was not like theirs. I listened to these comments and took them to heart; they kept me off my meds on more than one occasion. Deep down inside, I knew I loved the Lord. I trusted and believed in His will and healing power, maybe more so for others than for myself. And if being "saved" meant that I would have to suffer, I decided that I would.

Many Years Later

When I met my husband it was well after Mr Handsome had died. I missed him so much and prayed for God to send a man like him or better. When my husband came along, he was strongly built, big, and dark-skinned just like Mr. Handsome, and he even had the SAME first name; so I just knew my prayers were being answered and not soon after we married.....just like that!

Mr Handsome did not smoke, drink, or curse but my husband oh yes he did it all. And, no, it was not hidden, he didn't pretend to be a "new" creature around me. He was who he was at the very start but I'd told myself that God was going to deliver him because he promised me a husband and here he was even with the same name, come on now—I was sold!

Minister Mason and Mother Givhan both told me, "LeShaun, that is not your husband, baby. You're just believing what you want to believe and you can't hear anything else! When I married my husband, my thoughts were like that of all new brides. I wanted to live happily ever after. I desired to have a beautiful home, nice cars, and plenty of babies. Well, unfortunately, I had the pleasure of none of these.

For a season, intimacy with my husband was as painful as someone stabbing me with a pitch fork. I loved my husband and though we had problems in our marriage, sex was not one of them. I was a wife and I did all I knew to do to be a good wife. I prayed for my husband, putting his needs before my own, cooking, cleaning, being an ear and a shoulder to cry on. And yes putting his needs before my own when I was in pain.

He could not understand my pain and thought that I was making it up because I did not want to be with him. He even thought that I may have been sleeping with someone else, which I was not. Finally, I made a decision to see my doctor, who in turn scheduled me for tests, one of which was a laparoscopy. As she and another doctor whom she called into the room were looking at the screen and talking to each other, they began to explain to me their findings. My doctor said, "LeShaun, you have one, two, three, four, five fibroid tumors and severe endometriosis."

I asked, "What does all this mean?"

"This is why there is so much pain during intercourse and during your regular menstrual cycle," she said.

"What does this mean?" I asked again.

She replied, "The tumors are tightly attached to your ovaries and the endometriosis and damaged scar tissue from your abortions have severely damaged your uterus. I am recommending a hysterectomy."

"No!" I shouted. As I sobbed uncontrollably, my husband held my hand and tried comforting me by saying, "Baby, it's okay; we have Jazz."

But, I knew in his heart he wanted a biological child because we often discussed it and, I wanted more than anything to be able to give my husband a child. I could not believe it.

As many times as I had become pregnant, in sin and out of the will of God, this was not real. I could not help but think that I am saved , living as righteous as I knew how and married, why would this happen to me? I was everything that I should be now but unable to have a baby by my husband" I was devastated! At that time, I remembered God's Word:

> *Be not deceived; God is not mocked: for whatsoever a man soweth, that shall he also reap. For he that soweth to his flesh shall of the flesh reap corruption; but he that soweth to the Spirit shall of the Spirit reap life everlasting.*
>
> Galatians 6:7-8, KJV

This was one of the first things that came to mind. Was it hard? Yes, but it being a hard pill to swallow does not make the Word untrue and it is true not just for me but for all who live a reckless life.

Knowing how badly he wanted children, I gave up in my heart. I didn't think he could love me through it and I started thinking he was young enough to go have children with someone else. We both thought we were being everything we needed to be for and to one another. Being that it was our first marriage and we really didn't fight to stay together, we gave up. We may not have been young in age but mentally we were. And we moved faster than we should have in getting married. I took the time to just reflect on that memory and decided that this consecration was also healing me from the hurt of divorce. Then God continued working in me.

Spirit, Spirits, and More Spirits

These forty days of mirrors kept me on pins and needles. I really didn't know what God would flash before me next. Would it be a clear, clean mirror or one clouded and gray? Then, God revealed the **_anger_** that had settled within me. The scripture is very clear about anger:

> In your anger do not sin: Do not let the sun go down while you are still angry, and do not give the devil a foothold (a place from which an advance is made, like a military operation).
>
> Ephesians 4:26 -27

I allowed the spirit of anger to control my thoughts, moods, and actions. There was just so much that I felt I had a right to be angry about. I was angry because I felt my mother didn't support me. I was angry that my dad shunned me and did not show me any love. I was angry that it seemed as though my family favored my sister

71

over me. But most of all, I was angry at myself; because I realized that I could not make them love me and see good things in me. I was just angry all the time! But another scripture pointed out:

> *Know this, my beloved brothers: let every man be quick to hear, slow to speak, slow to anger; for the anger of a man does not produce the righteousness of God.*
> *James 1:19 -20, ESV*

I carried anger in my heart for so long that I thought God just didn't want anything to do with me. I felt that way because I could not understand why the fullness of God was not manifesting in my life. I also could not comprehend the overwhelming sense of anxiety that I dealt with on a daily basis. I truly thought it was God who had abandoned me because anger had occupied such a huge place in my heart. But eventually, I realized that it wasn't God but it was me!

> *Do not be anxious about anything, but in everything, by prayer and petition, with thanksgiving, present your request to God.*
> *Philippians 4:6, NIV*

The Spirit of Anxiety

My anxiety started as a little girl. I was always scared or worried about what I did, how I did it, and how much trouble I would get in before anything was ever said. Not that I was doing anything wrong at the time, but having seldom received praises for doing anything right caused me to always try harder to be something that I was not. I would do whatever it took to prove to you that I was good. I always believed that at some point I was going to do something wrong. I was always awaiting the next devastation, anticipating the next disaster, when by all accounts there was none.

This concentration forced me to look back and think things over. As a result, I had to stop and really thank God for where I am today. I am more complete now than I have ever been and it's because I made a choice to obey His instructions during this season of mirrors which He gently led me through. For forty days, I was truly seeing myself.

Back-biting and Gossip

God also dealt with me about something that so many of us have to confront and get out of our lives: that old spirit of back-biting and gossip. Backbiting is to speak unfavorably or slanderously behind the back of someone when they are not present, while gossiping is idle talk about the personal or private business of others.

At first, I really did not see this as an issue for me. When the mirror came before me and I looked through it, I can see situations where good people opened themselves to me and shared their innermost secrets and I unknowingly and knowingly betrayed them. At the time, I thought I was doing well by sharing information about others that was privately disclosed to me, especially when I thought it would help somebody else. However, many times it turned out to be a mess. I later began to see the revelation that when I was entrusted with information and told one person, it was an act of betrayal and I had failed.

I was at work, a male co-worker came to my desk chit chatting and flirting as usual. I looked at him and said, "I heard you were just a big womanizer who chased all sorts of women." He said, "Well, I heard you were messy, but that didn't stop me from trying to talk to you." Brining back those words at this time of my consecration truly made me search myself!

Standing Up For Right

Over time, I came to realize that it was so much easier to conform to the world's way and system than to be separated and come out from among them. Many times, it was easier to hear a smart or ugly comment about someone, listen, or even join in, rather than standing up and saying, "That is not right." You see, I learned that sometimes, standing up for "right" isolates you. It can make the world and even people who say they are Christians and serve the same God as you, dislike you. But, the Word of God states:

Am I now trying to win the approval of human beings or of God? Or am I trying to please people? If I were still trying to please people, I would not be a servant of Christ.

Galatians 1:10, NIV

"He says, she says, they say!" Does it really matter in the grand scheme of things? For me, I decided that it did not. I concluded that not standing up for what is right brings no glory to God. And at the end of the day I never want to bring shame, distrust, or lack of confidence to the Body of Christ, the ministry, and most importantly God Himself. When I recognized my part in not standing up for right, I cried out to God for forgiveness. In that moment, with tears running down my face, I heard God say this "You are loved by ME, called by ME, chosen by ME, and will be greatly used by ME. I have the first and final say according to my plan for your life! Now go and be blessed!"

Struggling with Church

I remember attending a church and being counseled by Minister Mason She was the one person able to make me open up and search my heart just by posing the simplest questions. At that time she helped me to recognize that in order to understand myself, I had to be willing to deal with and confront myself. For that I am grateful to God, because He used her at that time to start me on my journey of understanding and self-revelation.

When I came to know the Lord, (again not just going to church, but truly walking in the understanding of who He really is) I realized I was very naïve.. I was naïve when it came to understanding the Body of Christ, often referred to as the saints. I honestly believed that everyone was saved for real, delivered and set free from the ways of the world. I quickly discovered I was wrong. I learned that transitioning from the world to the church was not hard at all, because just like the world, you are surrounded by people who are hurting emotionally, mentally and spiritually. In the church, there are people carrying bitterness, anger, hurts, and unforgiveness. There are people, like me, needing approval and walking in that silent killer of the soul: depression.

Even though I was in the church and searching for God's will, I still felt the need to please people at the same time. I began serving in any area I could in order to show my gifts and gain the approval of others. I would find myself working with the youth, armor bearing, cooking, coordinating events, and more. Anything I could do to satisfy that little girl inside of me that needed to hear, "LeShaun, great job!" I have been in so many different churches seeking and searching for that one thing that the Lord was willing to give me freely: unconditional LOVE! I was broken, insecure, and bound with no real revelation of God's love for me. On account of this, the same sins, tricks, and lies that so easily beset me in the world, found me right in the church!

Many, many years ago, I met a man, an ordained elder, gifted in song and could preach and teach something serious. Yet, he was secretly sleeping with me! I knew I couldn't continue to do this, going to church on Sunday mornings, watching him lead praise and worship, encouraging the Saints to trust God and steer away from sin, and yet he had just left my home not thirty minutes earlier. And, he was planning on being there later that night. He never wanted us to arrive at the church at the same time. He didn't want us seen together as a couple. And, even though he treated me like that, I still chose to answer the door and the phone when he called.

I often wonder what drove me to get into all of the situations I would find myself in. Perhaps it was the musician who could play you into an anointed Holy Ghost-filled shout for hours, while yet sleeping with me and half the women in the church. Maybe it was the idea planted by the young lady who wanted to know if I was sleeping with the Pastor, because she was! Or, maybe it was the deacon that welcomed himself to my home unannounced. In fact, I will never forget that situation.

My daughter and I had been out of church, so the deacon from the church kept calling to "check" on us. I wasn't answering his calls, so he decided to show up at my house. He came in and urged me to come and sit by him on the couch, which I did not. Then upon him leaving, realizing that he was not getting anywhere with me, he stood at the door waiting for a "brotherly-sisterly" goodbye hug. As I leaned in to hug him he put one hand on each of my butt cheeks, squeezed and said, "If you only knew how bad I want you!" When he let me go, he was so stunned by my lack of response that fear came over him. I could tell from the look on his face that he realized he had done something wrong.

He asked me if he had offended me. By this time, I thought I had seen and heard everything concerning ministry, but I had not. I told him, "You have offended God and your wife more than you have offended me." I assured him that as for me telling the pastor or his wife, God would reveal his behavior to them in his time and season. That was the last time I heard from him. It is sad to say, but sexual sin still runs rampant in the church today. But I decided long ago to stop trying to keep myself and let Jehovah Adoni, the restorer of my soul and the true deliverer of all things, keep my mind, soul, and my body. You see, it was me all along. Some residue of my worldly ways was still there; whether I wanted to believe it or not, it was there even in my attempt to justify my actions by telling myself that I am this way because this or that happened to me.

Let us DISCERN FOR OURSELVES what is right;
let us learn together what is good!

Job 34:4, NIV

A very dear friend and I were discussing sexual perversion and how to better understand where it comes from. I shared with him my belief that some sexual perversion is birthed from sexual abuse, molestation, or other immoral acts if you will! Personally, the molestation I experienced opened doors in the area of sexual perversion and now, as an adult, I understand why and where the root of it came from. I also talked about how my experience with a woman at age fifteen was not a lesbian spirit for me, but it was a spirit of lust and sexual desires that overrode the fact that I was committing it with a woman.

Like getting high, the spirit of lust will make you feel like it's the best thing in the world and you just cannot get enough. When I got high, I did not care how big or small the joint was. I did not care if the weed was light green or dark green. I didn't care if the sheet I rolled the weed in was a fresh, unwrinkled sheet or an old ,wrinkled one out of my purse. I wanted that high and it didn't matter what package it came in! That's exactly how I felt with the spirit of lust. Oftentimes, it's not a physical attraction to a gender, but a sexual attraction to an act, at least that's what it was for me.

Therefore, when I realized that sexual high I received from a woman I could receive from a male, I then choose to stick with a male! There was a seed of sexual perversion and lust that was planted in my spirit when I was molested beginning at eight years of age. As a child, I was fighting sexual lust, perversion, and did not know it was wrong or even what to do about it! I desired to feel that way all the time in order to win other people's approval or affection.

I am learning to trust God to help me not give in to the advances of those who may be in the church, but the church is not in them. I am learning to guard myself from those who prey on innocent people like me. People who come from the world to the church seeking a real relationship with God but getting caught up in everything but. I am learning to focus on Jesus and the sacrifice He made on the cross for me, more than focusing on myself. This consecration kept showing seasons of my life that I truly needed deliverance from, so I learned to write down prayers and read them when I couldn't find the words.

Prayer

Dear God,

Please help me to deal with all the lions, bears and Goliaths in my life. Continue to strengthen me with your power so that I may be able to handle everything that comes my way. Not just handle things, but handle them the way Jesus would, with integrity and great character. Strengthen me to be able to endure, empower me with your power and make my desire to pray stronger. Your word tells me in 1 Peter 2:2, As newborn babies desire the sincere milk of the Word that I may grow thereby. My desire is to grow closer to You through Your word, so that I may be able to hear Your voice clearly, obey Your word, and be obedient to Your will for my life. I so desire peace in every area of my life. Have Your way in me. In Jesus name, Amen!

Your Daughter!

Church! For What?

From as early as I can remember, I was in church. Sunday School, Bible study, and Sunday morning services were all a part of my weekly life. As I grew older, I saw church as just another place to go. I knew of God, but I did not know God for myself. Fearing God was easier than obeying Him. I had been under the grace and mercy of a God who loved me raw and uncut, but I had no idea how to love Him back. Deep down in my heart, I knew that there was a work that the Lord God wanted me to do, but my impatience and disobedience in His direction for my life caused me to continue to walk in error. I often ask myself, how can I not serve a God that loves me so? A God who builds, grows, and prepares us for greatness even when we disobey Him. Only a good God would do that!

I honestly thought I was giving God my best when I chose to club, smoke weed, and fornicate before dragging myself to church Sunday morning. However, little did I know, I wasn't even close and a change in one of my friend's life would surely prove that.

After coming to a crossroad of change in her life, my friend, Donna, was determined to grow in God by any means necessary. She had come to a place where she decided that she did not want to continue going to church just for the sake of going. She desired a true encounter with Jesus Christ for herself, and she received it! Upon receiving Jesus as her Lord and Savior, she shared her experience with me!

Just as if it were yesterday, I can remember that season vividly. Donna's church was having a weeklong revival. Every day she would ask me, as we sat on our adjoining porches, if I would go to revival with her. She would say, "Ms. Taylor, you coming to church with me tonight?" I would raise my beer, blunt, or both and say, "Naw, Boo, but pray for me!" Her response to me was,

"Ok, momma, I got you!" Then the next night as she was on her way to revival, she would ask again, and I gave her the same answer.

On the last night of the revival, Donna asked again, "Ms. Taylor, you coming to church with me tonight?" This time, although the question was the same, my answer was different. I said "Yes." And that evening, I finished my beer, changed clothes, and went with her to church.

A New Desire

Church was not a new experience for me, but going there with the desire to feel God's true presence was. I can remember going up to the front of the church and humbling myself at the altar. I will never forget that moment. I felt the love of God cover me and my knees buckled as I hit the floor. The prayers that were going up, the spiritual language going forth by the people of God in other tongues, and the Glory that filled the place were simply wondrous! I wanted more.

When I left that night, I was filled and overwhelmed with a zest and zeal to know and experience more of God for myself. However, the more of God I desired, the more I realized that Satan desired me even the more! But, I went above and beyond to pursue righteousness. Even when I fell, or experienced shortcomings, I chased God with even more passion. The more I pursued God, the more I was willing to accept who I really wanted to become.

When I finally accepted Jesus as my Lord and Savior, I thought that I was instantly going to be delivered from sin. I said to myself, "Now, all is well and the devil will leave me alone." That thought was nowhere near the truth! We are talking about the devil. He held on as tight as he could to my life. So, the thought that he would let me go and leave me alone that easily was a HOT mess!

In reality, he left me alone for a season. But then, he would come back with an attack greater than the last one. My fights with him were always messy. Unfortunately, I would always end up defeated because I did not know how to fight a spiritual battle. In the midst of these messy fights, I would always remember this scripture:

> *For our struggle is not against flesh and blood, but against the rulers, against the authorities, against the powers of this dark world and against the spiritual forces of evil in the heavenly realms. Therefore put on the full armor of God, so that when the day of evil comes, you may be able to stand your ground, and after you have done everything, to stand.*
>
> *Ephesians 6:12-13, NIV*

I had heard this scripture many times in my life. I quoted it never having any real revelation of it and never having no authority when quoting it. I was fighting people, things, and situations. I was always wrestling with flesh and blood. I never understood that the fight was not against people, but it was against the spirits of the evil one.

Backsliding....
Oh Yes, That was definitely me!

"Your wickedness will punish you; your backsliding will rebuke you. Consider me and realize how evil and bitter it is for you when you forsake the Lord your God and have no awe (emotion caused by something extraordinary) of me" declares the Lord, the Lord Almighty.

Jeremiah 2:19, NIV

I sat in this period of consecration with God reflecting all of me back to my true self. I didn't want to take any more notes, write any more names, or read any more scriptures. I was counting down the days to end this. But the mirrors God revealed continued to show me more of my self. At this point I started to understand that my backsliding always occurred when I was overwhelmed and isolated. It would hit me when I had given up on myself and abandoned all hopes of God rescuing me out of my current circumstance. It would happen when my faith had dwindled and I had lost all hope and trust. I would look for people, places, cities, men, alcohol, and even cigarettes to fill the void I felt inside. In thinking through this, the Holy Spirit released a scripture to encourage my soul:

> *Turn, O backsliding children, saith the LORD; for I am married unto you: and I will take you one of a city, and two of a family, and I will bring you to Zion:*
>
> *Jeremiah 3:14*

As I continued to grow in my relationship with the Lord, His grace kept me when I stumbled. He never allowed me to fall beyond the reach of His hand. That same grace picked me back up again and again. I sincerely repented, dusted myself off, and continued my pursuit of God. One of my greatest desires birthed out of my communion with God was to be filled with the Holy Ghost with the evidence of speaking in new tongues and have God's power to cast out demons. Although I had been baptized in water as a child and as an adult, I desired all the blessings that came with being a believer according to scripture:

He said to them, "Go into all the world and preach the good news to all creation. Whoever believes and is baptized will be saved, but whoever does not believe will be condemned.And these signs will accompany those who believe: In my name they will drive out demons; they will speak in new tongues; they will pick up snakes with their hands; and when they drink deadly poison, it will not hurt them at all; they will place their hands on sick people, and they will get well."

Mark 16: 15-18, NIV

After reading this scripture, my desire to serve God heightened!

A Desire Only He Could Give

Several years later, I met a sister in the Lord who was not just on fire for God, but her servanthood to Him and people was absolutely awesome! I shared with her my desire to serve God, even in the mist of the mess that I was yet being delivered from. In my heart, I really wanted to be used of God. One night this young lady invited me to her home for Bible study and prayer. As she opened with prayer, she asked God to give us clarity and understanding of His Word. After we studied the rich word of God, she told us that we would close the evening in prayer, but before we prayed, she wanted to offer some instructions. She told us to ask God for a desire that only He could give. She also said that after we prayed, we would take some time to worship God.

As we began to pray, I eagerly began petitioning God, asking the Holy Spirit to fill me with His presence. All of a sudden, I started crying and screaming uncontrollably. At first, I was embarrassed and ashamed because I felt as though I could not stop myself. I began throwing up, shaking, and stammering. Then all of a sudden, I was speaking in other tongues (a language God inspired that is different than my native language). This was the beautiful baptism of the Holy Ghost. It was one of the most awesome experiences of my life.

Now, you would think that I was totally free from my past, fleshly desires and cravings after that experience, but I was not. For many years that followed, I continued to wrestle with fornication and bouts of uncontrolled depression. However, it was only when I opened myself up to truly understand God's word, His will for my life, and gave Him a total "Yes" from the bottom of my heart, that I was able to see where the attacks of the enemy really came from the invisible spirit realm.

Low self-esteem, depression, suicidal thoughts, insecurities, rebellion, anger, and bitterness, just to name a few, are all demonic spirits that can only be fought by the higher, more powerful Spirit. Yes, that Spirit is the Holy Spirit—the Spirit of God—the undefeated champion of the universe!

But you will receive power when the Holy Spirit comes on you; and you will be my witnesses in Jerusalem, and in all Judea and Samaria, and to the ends of the earth."

Acts 1:8, NIV

The Spirit of Fear

The spirit of fear kills your hopes, steals your visions, and destroys the will and purpose of God in your life. I had allowed the spirit of fear to cripple my walk with God and hinder my growth. Although I wanted to blame others, I realized at some point I could not.

Nightmares, phobias, anxiety, stress, double mindedness, intimidation, fear of failure, and fear of persecution, I'd always grappled with them. They are demonic spirits, and even until this day some have been harder to fight than others. I had been in bondage to these demonic forces by choice for most of my life. I was choosing to believe Satan's lies instead of God's truth about me. I was choosing to be the tail and not the head because of fear; fear that I am not truly all that God says I am. I would soak up the lies that were said about me and even more damaging, I would believe the lies that I would tell myself about myself. The root source of all of this comes from FEAR. The Bible states:

For God hath not given us the spirit of fear; but of power, and of love, and of a sound mind.

2 Timothy 1:7

Intimidation and Insecurity

I had a revelation that really amazed and freed me at the same time. The revelation was to simply "Stop calling everybody mister and ma'am." I thought, "Ok, God, I will obey, but how is that one of my issues? What category have I put that under?" He said, "Intimidation and insecurity." Instead of using these titles as a sign of respect or good manners as taught by many people, I would use them to reference or attribute peoples' position, importance, or even their spiritual callings to be superior to mine.

I was very insecure. I never thought what I had to say mattered, let alone was valued. If anything, I was always considered the Drama Queen or the Simpleton, so it was easy for me to stoop down and allow others to stand on my shoulders or even my face. I had no problem being intimidated or seeing others in a greater light than what God's word said about me.

I never believed in my heart that God could or would use me like He used my awesome, anointed friends. I felt their favor, grace and level of knowledge in the things of God was always greater than my own. I would even allow the world to trick me in that same manner. I would find myself giving excessive honor and respect to men and women who were not even sons and daughters of God because I felt that even in their sinful state, they were more worthy than I. I took what God was revealing and waited a few moments, knowing that He would soon bring back to my memory examples of the behavior He was working to free me from. God's personality began to become clearer as this consecration continued.

Servant or a Maid?

Sure enough, the memory came. One day after church, several of our church members and I had gathered to fellowship at the home of my friend Justin, a gifted man of God whose wisdom and knowledge I trusted. I love to cook and serve people, so that's what I was busy doing. After we had eaten and everyone was seated in the living room discussing how rich the Word was at church that morning. As the conversation continued, guess where I was? In the kitchen washing dishes, drying them, and putting them away. The man of God, my friend Justin, stood up and said, "If you don't get out of that kitchen and come in here with us, you ain't a maid!"

That incident was brought back to my remembrance. The Lord said to me "There is a difference between having a servant's heart and being subservient." That knocked blew my mind! A servant is someone who performs household or personal duties, housekeeper, butler, etcetera. They receive pay, yet they still have a servant's heart because of their gifting to be useful and helpful to others. A pastor can have a servant's heart because of his calling and love for people, and his desire to render obedience and homage to God.

God explained, "You had neither. You, daughter, were just a slave." A slave is considered the property of another person, a person who does very hard or dull work, someone who devotes serious efforts to something because they are subservient. To be subservient means to serve or act in a lowly or subordinate capacity. I realize that I had been a slave to other people's opinion of me. A slave to approval and acceptance, a slave to hurt, bitterness and anger! I thought on what this invisible, mighty God was showing me and I was overwhelmed with emotions so deep I felt the correction. Later that night, I read these scriptures:

> *"It is for freedom that Christ has set us free. Stand firm, then, and do not let yourself be burdened again by a yoke of slavery."*
>
> *Galatians 5:1, NIV*

Jesus replied, "I tell you the truth, everyone who sins is a slave to sin. Now a slave has no permanent place in the family, but a son belongs to it forever. So if the Son sets you free, you will be free indeed.

John 8:34-36, NIV

Choices

Life is choice driven. At that time, I chose not to walk in freedom, but rather to succumb to fear, insecurity and intimidation. I chose slavery.... I realized that fear, insecurity, and intimidation were generational curses in my life. These phobias aided in destroying my relationships and had the potential to affect my daughter and generations after her. So, I rebuked that devil and I prayed.

Prayer

Strongman, otherwise known as the spirit of fear and bondage, you will not have my children or the generations that will come through their wombs. Anything attached to them through the bloodline, or in the air in which you happen to be prince of, is cancelled in Jesus' name. The curse is broken with me and will not touch my daughters and beyond! Jesus bore it all on the cross for me and for generations to come! Amen!

Your Daughter

God explained that all of those spirits are based out of the spirit of fear and from fear came the spirit of rejection. For me rejection by people, as well self-rejecting, came from a feeling of worthlessness. I knew God was trying to bring comfort in clarifying my feelings, but I was surrounded by conviction and ready for the consecration to end.

With this in mind, we constantly pray for you, that our God may count you worthy of his calling, and that by his power he may fulfill every good purpose of yours and every act prompted by your faith.

2 Thessalonians 1:11, NIV

Over the years, I have had many awesome people speak of Gods awesomeness into my life, sharing with me Gods promises and that He is no respecter of person, He loves us ALL and wants His best for each of us. I remember not feeling my best and wanting a Word clearly from God for me. Justin and Patrica heard that a great and mighty woman of God was speaking at a church about two to three hours outside of where we lived and I was ready to go.

My prayer was "God, please let me hear a Word especially for me. I don't know how you are going to do it but please do it for me. Well, when I tell you God will do it. We had gotten to the church and praise and worship had just started. Then the woman of God came out in the mist of us praying and started to pray with us. Then she began to minister and the atmosphere for worship was ever present. I couldn't put my hands down or stop crying. But I could hear her talking. I could hear her moving around and suddenly, I heard her say, "Move, move, move over! I'm trying to get to her!'" With my hands raised in worship, I'm thinking, *Lord, bless whoever she is trying to get to.* Then, I felt warm hands on my forehead. "Yesssssssss!" She screamed As I fell to the ground crying, she started speaking into my life, "God has destined you for great things but you are always waring in your mind; you've never believed God could do anything for you! Your battlefield is in your mind!" She shouted, "Be set free and TRUST GOD's plan for your life!"

She walked away from me, leaving a plush, ten-foot purple towel to cover me. She walked from person to person, blessing their lives. Then, I heard her again, "Move, move let me get down there with her!" She continued to bless my life more by speaking power, binding up the spirit of low self-esteem, saying, "There are things you deal with in your mind that have tried to take you out of here!" And I'm on the floor of the sanctuary balling, tears flowing everywhere.

It was an awesome service from beginning to end. My friends kept teasing me, "How she gone move us out the way to get to you?" But, I knew and God knew and when I shared my testimony with them what I had prayed for that day: for God to give me a direct and *right now* Word and for me to know it was Him, they were in awe and all the Saints could say was, "YES, WONT HE DO IT !"

Hurt Caused, Hurt Endured

Sometime later, after seeing several doctors and coming to a resolve of really trying to be off of the meds, God would use one of my doctors to show Himself to me, to show me that He cared about everything that concerned me. Dr. K became such a blessing to me in both natural and spiritual things. One day, Dr. K said to me, "LeShaun, you carry so much hurt and guilt. If you were Catholic, I would tell you to get an absolution." I looked at her curiously.

An absolution is a formal release from guilt. It is a pronouncement of forgiveness that is made after a person has repented to a priest. This religious rite is centered on the forgiveness that Jesus extended to sinners during his ministry. In the early church, the priest would absolve repentant sinners after they had confessed and performed a penance in public. Dr. K continued, "You need to know that God does not hold on to all those things from your past. The hurt you have endured and the hurt you have caused have all been forgiven It is not God's will for you to live condemned for the rest of your life!"

I finally met a doctor who said, "You are not crazy and taking medication does not make you love God any less." She explained that I had a chemical imbalance which came about through no fault of my own. For me, that explanation was so liberating. It gave me the ability to be at peace about getting the help I needed and deserved. As a result of her truthfulness and gentle guidance, I've taken my medication for bipolar disorder faithfully! And as I continue to seek a full deliverance from God, I will take it until deliverance comes! Just as a diabetic or someone with high blood pressure takes medicine, I take medicine for a diagnosed illness. What I have learned through this struggle is that there often is no end-all or be-all quick cure to anything. However, today I can say that I have never felt freer to be who God created me to be than I do now! I am an heir to the Kingdom of God!

There is surely a future hope for you, and your hope will not be cut off.

Proverbs 23:18, NIV

Prayer

Father, I thank you. I thank You because no matter what it looks like around me, You assure me that my future is filled with hope and that it will not be cut off, no matter who or what! I am grateful that You are teaching me that I must learn to change my daily confessions from defeat and doubt to victory and triumph over all situations that may come my way. I must trust You, God; not just in word, but in action, lifestyle, and through spoken word. God, please help me to trust You like I never knew I could. Please show me Your will for my life, and make Your will clear.

Your Daughter

Bearing It All

This consecration left me drained. But it also left me feeling liberated. My teenage daughter watched me struggle those forty days. She heard my cries. She really saw the seriousness of this consecration on the eighteenth day. She was cooking fish and I thought, *Lord, I have been faithful I don't think a small taste will hinder my growth at this point.* Not thirty minutes later, the side of my face grew two sizes and Jazzy was rushing me to the Emergency Room. It was painful! I cried and repented all the way there. Once checked in and taken to a back room, the doctor came in baffled saying, "We will run a few tests, but you may be allergic to seafood." I said, "Doctor, I have been eating seafood all of my life, that can't be it." Then my daughter said, "She not allergic to seafood. She's allergic to disobedience. There is no medicine that can fix disobedience!" She witnessed this process and basically said if you are going to go in and do this fast, go to the end.

Often times when things are going well we can allow ourselves to be deceived into thinking that we have everything under control. I know, because when I thought I didn't need to be kept, I deliberately chose to walk from under the covering and blessings of God. Please do not misunderstand me, I wanted to be blessed, but there was still that part of me that wanted to do what I wanted to do as well. Just like the story of the prodigal son who chose to get his inheritance from his father early and leave from under the protection and covering of His Father's house to do what he wanted to do (Luke 15:11-32), I too walked away from under God's perfect will for my life to do what I wanted to do. I wanted to do, go, and see what I wanted to, and I wanted to do those things exactly how I wanted. And it has been those "I wants" that have always gotten me in trouble!

Divine Revelations

During the consecration and after, I learned and I am still learning so much about the me God sees. It has truly been a journey of self-reflection and discovery. It is my prayer that it will be the same for you.

It is never easy sharing all of your sins, past or present, to an audience of people you may or may not know. I am choosing to share to let people know that God is a healer. For me, I had to release sexual, spiritual, mental and emotional soul ties. Even though I was no longer involved with any of them, I felt that they would always have a tie to me if I allowed them to do so. But, I prayed a prayer of release and now I no longer believe that. Therefore, if you have had or still have some of the challenges you can pray this payer, and believe it in your heart, and God will set you free. He did it for me, and He will do the same for you!

The Continuation

God continues to show me things about myself that years ago I would not have received or believed. I could receive it about you, but not about me. I started asking myself questions, but the most significant one was, "Are you saying you have it all together now?" The answer is no. In myself I don't, but I have a God who not only has it ALL together, but who knows how to get me together at the same time.

Today, I am ever learning, ever growing, and ever yearning for the meat of God's word. I know that I truly need the word of God, the blood of Jesus, and the grace of God to keep me. To seal this revelation, God gave me an absolutely clear analogy! Now, we do know that God is loving, kind, all powerful, all knowing and His wrath is mighty; but, he is also humorous!

One morning, I was on the couch half asleep and awake, when the Lord showed me mini clips of the cartoon Charlie Brown. The Lord showed me the character Pig-Pen and said clearly, "Don't let this be you!" I opened one eye, looked around and then opened the other thinking, Seriously God, Pig-Pen! Pig-Pen was the one who simply could not stay clean, no matter what. It seemed that even after many attempts at cleaning himself up; he was dirty all over again. Then I thought, Lord the dust and dirt that Pig-Pen experienced were all outward. He was, as I recall, a good kid. Then the Lord led me to look up the word dirt and this is what I found:

Final Revelations

Dirt–(noun)

1. Any foul or filthy substance, as mud, grime, dust, or excrement. Something or someone vile, mean, or worthless: After that last outburst of hers I thought she was dirt.

1. moral filth; vileness; corruption.

1. or lewd language: to talk dirt.

1. Informal. gossip, esp. of a malicious, lurid, or scandalous nature: Tell me all the latest dirt.

1. private or personal information which if made public would create a scandal or ruin the reputation of a person, company, etc.

1. Mining.

a.   crude, broken ore or waste.

a. (in placer mining) the material from which gold is separated by washing.

—Idioms

    2. do (someone) dirt. Dirty (def. 18).

1.   eat dirt, Informal . to accept blame, guilt, criticism, or insults without complaint; humble or abase oneself: The prosecutor seemed determined to make the defendant eat dirt.

My first thought was how can that be me? I have consecrated before you, repented, and been in much prayer and now this? I began to think back to the issues that caused me to throw my hands up in the first place. Those things that caused me to say, "HELP me, Lord. I am sick and tired of myself, the filth, the guilt, even the smell of me." I came to the realization that sin stinks and when you walk in it, wallow in it, and wander around it, you began to reek the horrendous smell of it.

Even after I consecrate, fast and pray, I have to remember those things that caused me to fall in the first place. The stench that attached itself to me: rebellion, fornication, gossip, low self-esteem insecurities, hurt, bitterness; all that dirt can only be cleared and cleansed by continual prayer and fasting, continual crying out to God, and continual yearning to walk in and remain free!

I realized that the strongest, most lathered up, best-selling soap won't wash away the stench of sin. My Jesus! Not even the hottest of showers will be able to take away the things that reek from within and seeps out. Only the blood of Jesus, the desire for true revelation of self and a willingness to walk out the deliverance process at any cost can and will send a sweet smelling fragrance that will please God! Thank you to the King of Kings for taking me from being Pig-Pen to being an heir to the throne of Jehovah Elyon…The Lord Most High! What he did, and continues to do for me, He can do for you!

Prayer

Father God, in the name of Jesus, I thank You this day. For it is a day of supernatural release from every person, place, or thing that has attached itself to or that has tied itself to my life. God, thank You for delivering me from every demonic spirit, force, fruit, and lie that has come through generational bloodlines and personal sexual contact; be it intercourse, oral sex, kissing, fondling, phone sex, and sexual conversation. God, I confess and release unto to You, this day, everyone who I have come into contact with in a sexual, lustful, emotional, spiritual, and mental way. I ask and I thank you for releasing me from them and them from me in the name of Your son Jesus Christ, and by His blood. Lord, thank You that every hindering spirit that stops Your will from manifesting itself in my life is bound. As I look back and think, I give all of the sexual or immoral situations that have happened in my life over to you along with any fornicating, adultery, masturbation, oral sex, lust, lesbian, sodomy, pornography, molestation spirits, and sexual perversion of all kinds. Lord, I thank You that I am delivered and set free by Your Word, Your blood, and the confession of my faith, not in my ability, but in Yours and the work You finished on Calvary's Cross. Thank you Lord, In Jesus name I pray, Amen!

Your Daughter

The Me God Sees

I am a decade older at the publishing of this book. Learning more about God's Word and understanding myself has been my main objective. I can never thank God enough for growing me, building me and revealing me to me. I feel a freedom now that I have never felt in my life. I am learning to love me and I am seeing glimpses of "the me" God sees! No, I am not perfect; but, that is one of the things that has brought me more ease. There is none perfect but the Father!

I had spent all of my life trying to be someone who I was never purposed or ordained to be. I was trying to be perfect, pretending to have it all together, fronting like I was happy-go-lucky because any sign of failure or sadness brought shame upon me and the ministry of God! But, I have made a choice to live my life to its fullest without shame, guilt, or condemnation. How long will this last? I'm not sure, but I do know this, that God is yet revealing to me every day how beautiful I am to Him, and how beautiful I have always been!

The last couple of years have been more than a little challenging. I have experienced so many different things, such as leaving my home, my friends, my job to relocate to what I deemed to be the desert; my mom's sudden stroke; the death of one of my best friends; wrestling with bouts of depression; chasing jobs and hoop dreams; and the list goes on and on! But I will say this, even when I did not realize it, God had me, and yes He did! And what I have appreciated is that ALL things work out for the good of those who love the Lord, and I love the Lord!

I am walking in a new light and I have recently been able to look at my past with empathy and not so much anger and resentment! I am more together now than I was thirty, twenty, or even ten years ago! For me, that is a great thing because so many people leave this earth without ever getting it together or even desiring to get it together!

To everyone that has read this book and have shared this journey of discovery with me, I thank you for taking time to allow me to enter your heart and your thoughts. I pray that in some way I was able to enrich your life with my testimony. I pray that in some way I caused you to take a look inside of yourself and recognize your own demons, faults, failures judgments and criticisms and then being able to say, "You know what, it was me all along!" That doesn't negate from the fact that yes people hurt us, fail us, abuse us, talk about and deceive us. But, the truth of the matter is, if we are not careful we will continue to be victims by choice because it's easier to lie down and play dead rather than stand and fight! Fight for what, you ask? Fight for our healing, our sanity, and our purpose! God's plan for my life is not over. It is only just beginning.

God is making me over to be all that he has called me to be. Will I fall, will I trip up and slip up, and will I sometimes not get it right? Yes, but then I am reminded of this one thing:

> *A righteous man falleth seven times, and rises up again: but the wicked are over thrown by calamity"*
> *Proverbs 24:16 KJV*

I choose to rise up again, and again, and again, and again, and again and oh yes, again. I now choose to accept the bitter with the sweet. I choose to look at myself and say it is not my mother, my father, my sister, my aunt, uncle or cousin but it is me oh Lord, standing before you in the need of prayer for the things that I have done, whether knowingly or unknowingly.

Prayer

Forgive me, Lord for choosing to walk in unforgiveness, for choosing to walk in shame and condemnation, even when I knew better it was simply easier to walk in sorrow than to deal with myself!

Your Daughter

Just recently my doctor asked me, "LeShaun, are you starting to feel more like yourself?" I looked at her with such curiosity and I said, "You know Doc, I don't know if I really know what I am feeling. I have been so depressed, so sad, so angry, hurt and bitter for all my life. I don't know how the "real me" is supposed to feel.

At that moment, I realized that I had accepted myself the way I was and I did not bother to see or even care to know if there were better ways to feel. I never considered "the me" God sees. My health is better and so is my outlook on life. This precious life that God has given me is moving onward and upward! I remember many years ago my dear friend and mentor, Minister Mason, used to say, "Baby, you cannot always get the peace around you that you want, but you can always choose to have peace and rest on the inside of you and always remember who's for you....if God be.....!"

—Letters of Love and Gratitude—

God,

I can never thank You enough for Your unconditional love, unmerited grace, and unlimited mercy which supersede anything I could have ever done for myself. Even in the midst of my disobedience, disrespect, and dysfunction toward You, Father, You still continued to pour Your love upon me. You are my all. It has taken me all of my life to come to that conclusion. Because of who You are, I give You glory. Because of who You are, I give You praise. Because of who You are, I write this book in honor of You!

'

~~~~

Jazmin,

I write this book to share my tests and testimonies with you. You have been my inspiration and the reason I chose to be obedient in writing this memoir. Jazmin, you are such a beautiful child both inside and out. I remember when I first found out I was pregnant with you. I was so scared that I could not or would not be able to be all that you needed me to be as your parent. But as you grew inside of me, I knew God would equip, guide, and instruct me along the way. I started talking to you and singing the alphabet song to you at least ten times a day.

When I was given a stethoscope, I would spread the earpiece on each side of my belly and talk to you from the other end. I talked to you day in and day out. I continued to pray for the Lord to teach me all the skills needed to be a great parent to you. I would cry and say, "Lord, don't let Jazz have to endure the hurt and rejection that I had during my childhood and into my adulthood." I know we all have to experience some things for ourselves, but I didn't want you to have to endure not even a fourth of the things that I had endured. I can truly say God is faithful, and He does answer prayers.

Jazmin, no matter what happens from here on out, your strength, determination, and love have blessed my life in ways that mere words on paper can never fully express. You've always made sure I continued looking at the hills from where my help comes instead of looking at the rocks below, the bumps in the road, or even the green grass, but straight ahead, focusing on the promises of God.

I have fallen down on this journey of knowing, understanding, and loving myself so many times that there aren't enough fingers or toes on earth to keep up with the count. However, when I do fall into that unforeseen or sometimes seen pit, you reach your hand out and say, "Ma, come on." You have been more than a daughter to me, you have been my friend, my confidant, and—on many occasions—you have had to assume the role of mother!

At times, so much responsibility is placed on a child born of a mother who still deals with depression, unhealed hurts, and bleeding wounds. But the key word to that is "born." You were born of a mother not just because that is who I am to you. You were born because of who you are destined to be for God. I love you, yes, but God knew you before the foundations of the earth and purposed for you to come this way via me.

What a bright and promising future the Lord God has in store for you, Jazmin! In spite of all our dysfunction and chaos, you have grown up to be all that the Lord has promised and more. I am just as honored to have carried you, birthed you, and raised you as Mary was with Jesus. I am proud of you, your past, present, and the awesome future the Lord has divinely designed for you. I appreciate you, support you, encourage you, value you, thank you, and will always love you!

~~~~

Lady D,

I remember when we first met. You were somewhat shy, with beautiful eyes and tiny feet. Almost instantly you became my friend. Over our twenty-year friendship, there were many challenges, disagreements, and times of separation, but in spite of it all, our love for each other never wavered. You understood me with all my faults and shortcomings.

Donna, you were such a unique person. You loved, gave, and shared yourself with me and so many others.

When you were first diagnosed with cancer, we cried, uncertain of what it all meant for you, your future, and your son Justin. You worried less about the cancer and more about Justin who you were raising to be an awesome, God-fearing, and mature young man. You were a great mother, and with your diagnosis you took nothing for granted. From there, super mom arose. You began pouring out so much of you into Justin. You shared God, strength, honesty, loyalty, concerns, and your anointing with him.

I watched you become stronger than the rock that killed Goliath. Even during heartache, heartbreak, letdowns, disappointments, and hurt, you never once complained. You always wanted to know how Jazz and I were doing, even how my Mom, Lunda, and Oscar were doing. You wanted to make sure I was doing well. When I would ask, "Lady D, how are you feeling?" You would say, "Look here, lady. Don't worry about me. God has me!"

As we talked through years of hospital stays and chemotherapy, you always found ways to encourage and uplift me in Jesus. Your zeal never ceased to amaze me. Your motto was always "whatever the will of God is for me, I am in full agreement because I know it will work out for the good!" As time passed, you endured much physical pain, and I watched you soar above it all in your mind and spirit. You made a choice on how you were going to handle that demon called cancer and you chose to live!

Then one day my phone rang. You were on the other end telling me that Justin, your lil king who was nine at the time, had just been diagnosed with the same disease. As you cried uncontrollably, I could barely understand your words. However, I did hear you scream from the bottom of your belly, "Shaun, I don't want him to suffer! This is not supposed to happen to him!" You demanded that I pray for Justin like never before. I prayed and prayed as you and Justin grew closer to God and each other, learning and understanding more about the disease that had befallen you both. Justin has always been a special little boy, very curious. He did not mind asking questions and always wanted an answer. You answered those questions as best as you could and taught him right from wrong. You taught him about love, strength, and how to do others as he would want them to do him. And, my dear friend, sister, ace-boon-coon, and encourager, you succeeded!

Then, that day came. I remember lying on the floor at Shands Hospital holding your foot while they pulled the plug on your body. A body that had been ravaged by so much hurt, heartache, and pain, I listened to the moans of the people you left behind. I heard the sobs of your mother who deemed you not just her daughter, but her best friend and the love of her life. You meant so much to her that she didn't know how she would go on without you! I could hear your brother crying heartfelt tears of pain grieving the last breaths of his sister. You were his oldest sister. You not only loved him but could not have been more proud of him than if you had birthed him yourself. All of the friends and family, who remember your love, your strength, and your faithfulness to each of us, were grieving.

I assure you this, Justin has all the strength, power, and honor you wanted and more. You were so proud of him, but I don't think you were prouder of him than he was and still is of you! I write this book in your remembrance.

~~~~

Oscar,

What can I say about my Oscar, my only nephew? I love you so much, and I am proud of the man that God is shaping you to become. You have learned how to deal with all these women in your life. Our moods—okay, let me rephrase that, "my moods"—our way of thinking, and our out-of-the-box attitude. With God's guidance, your mom raised and nurtured you to be strong-minded, compassionate, and a wise young man beyond your years. I am so very excited about your future. From the time you were born, you were the "man of the house." There have been times when I have learned so much from you. You always give me advice straight up and on point, never wavering! When we get together as a family and conversations get a little heated, you would stand up and say, "Alright now, enough is enough" and a hush would come over the room because Big O had spoken. Your nature has always been to love us, protect us, listen to us, encourage us, and calm us all at the same time. For that I am ever so grateful. You, nephew, are my baby boy and I will love you unconditionally, always!

~~~~

Youlunda,

You have always been there for Mya, Jazzy, and me! I remember back to a conversation we had many years ago. You said, "You know, we really do not have much in common to be sisters." That statement has always stuck with me because no matter what we did, it seemed that we truly had nothing in common. But the more I thought about it, the more I realized that we actually did and still do have things in common. We love each other and want God's very best for each other. Although we have had many disagreements, laughter, weave follies (lol), and deep discussions, through them all we have been there for one another. You opened your home to a dysfunctional me on many occasions, allowing me and my baggage to invade your privacy and your private space. Until this day, I cannot remember you complaining once. And for that I give you a SUPER thank you, Sis!

~~~~

Mommy,

I remember watching you as a little girl, proud of all the things you achieved. You were always dreaming and believing for more. You not only dreamed it, you lived it to the best of the ability God had given you. When you opened your fashion studio many years ago, I was always in awe of you and the things you accomplished along the way. I loved helping you, even if it was just holding the pins and the tape measure around my neck. I remember watching your models. They were bold, beautiful, and extra tall (at least six feet or taller)! As a little girl, I watched them practice before a show, modeling clothes that you had created from scratch. To see your designs was inspiring, but to see them come to life on the runway was mesmerizing! I remember so clearly one instance where you were making a first time designer wedding gown. Watching your vision come to life as you connected one piece to another was sheer genius. When the moment arrived, the bride walked in looking radiant in not just a dress, but in a Taylor Doll original. At the reception, the bride started spinning in one spot, taking off pieces of the gown revealing another outfit underneath the gown. Mom, you did that. I can honestly say my creative juices and fire for seeing the unseen in visions and dreams came from you.

I remember us never missing the yearly fair that came to town. I re-member the parrot jungle, the dolphin shows at the aquarium, the Lion Country Safari, and so much more. You always availed yourself to us as children; nothing seemed to come before us. And then suddenly, you became a single parent. Your life shifted by no fault of your own, but that was the beginning of change for all of us.

Life's demands on you were great and you went to working only what I deemed as a few hours a day to working from sun up to sun down, literally! Maybe I was jealous, selfish, or rebellious but I didn't have you anymore.

In my mind, I was always awaiting this grand come back where you would continue to defy the odds and pursue your dreams and goals with due diligence. That never happened and in a way I was upset with you for not pushing for that "better" you always told us about. Helping you bus tables, clean rooms, and waitress was ideal because we were together; but I would always tell myself this is only temporary, this cannot be the end, there is so much greatness inside of my mom, and this cannot be how it ends.

Today, I realize this one thing that I have to love you where you are and not where I want you to be. I have learned that you have endured much suffering, and you are still here to tell the story. I have learned that being afflicted with a stroke is no match for you. You are a survivor, you are a winner. I was watching you walk the other day, going down the hall to play bingo with your friends, and I thought "simply amazing"! Being paralyzed has had an emotional and physical toll on you, but you wake up, get dressed, cook, wash clothes, and faithfully attend church. That little girl that was in awe of you so many years ago is now a grown woman, but she is still in awe of you and all that you do!
I love you, Ma!

~~~~

Daddy,

As I sit here, I ask the Lord to give me the words to share how I feel about our relationship. I wanted a way that would describe my heart to you! I was led back to a movie, "The Color Purple."

There were many scenes in this film where Shug, the rebellious, prodigal daughter, reached out to her father, the stubborn, no nonsense Pastor. There was the scene where she came to talk to him at the church. He was alone cleaning. As she approached, he sat down with his back to her listening to her plea. Shug just wanted a response of any kind out of him. But he just walked out of the sanctuary. Then there was the scene where Shug came outside to check the mail and she saw her father riding a carriage up the dirt road. She ran to him screaming, "Look, Daddy, I's married now! I's married now!" What she was saying is daddy look at me, am I now worthy of your love, attention and affection? Be proud of me please!

And up until that point in the movie I thought I had no more tears to cry, boy was I wrong! When Shug was at the juke joint singing and doing her thing, she hears the choir at her father's church singing "God is Trying to Tell You Something". She walked for what seemed like forever singing that song, making her way to the church. Shug arrived, singing from her gut like she had never done. She makes her way to the altar with tears in her eyes and she says, "See, Daddy, sinners have souls, too."

When her dad stepped down from the pulpit and embraced her, the weight of hurt, bitterness, and instability in her life and spirit was lifted. Just one embrace from the only man in her life that could make her feel whole made her feel more loved and worthy than ALL of the men who had come and gone in her life.

Well, Daddy, I await our "church house" moment. I await that life changing, memory-making, curse-breaking, past-forgiving embrace. I await the weight finally being lifted! You are my daddy and I love you, always and forever!

I am so grateful that we have both grown and matured. I never saw myself having weekly phone conversations but now we do. It means such so much to have grown past where we were for so many years of my life to this awesome new place. Thank you for spending holidays with me and my girls. I love you dearly!

~~~~

Pops and Mother Givhan,

Sometimes God puts people in your path to teach you, correct you, love you, and get you together all at the same time. You have been that to me. Your support throughout more than a decade of my life has enriched me. No matter the ups or the downs, and there were—okay, there are— many.

You never shunned me, discouraged me, or rejected me. They say some people are here for reasons, seasons, or lifetimes. Well, Jazmin, Mya, and I believe God for a prosperous, faithful, and healthy **LIFETIME!**

~~~~

I also thank you, the reader, for purchasing and supporting my very first literary work.

Thank you,
LeShaur

CPSIA information can be obtained
at www.ICGtesting.com
Printed in the USA
FFHW011536081219
56559499-62384FF